Speech/Language Therapists and Teachers Working Together

A Systems Approach to Collaboration

Speech/Language Therapists and Teachers Working Together

A Systems Approach to Collaboration

EDITED BY

ELSPETH MCCARTNEY

Department of Speech and Language Therapy,
Faculty of Education, University of Strathclyde

W

WHURR PUBLISHERS

LONDON

© 1999 Whurr Publishers Ltd

First published 1999
by Whurr Publishers Ltd
19b Compton Terrace
London N1 2UN
England,

Reprinted 2000

British Library Cataloguing in Publication Data
A catalogue record for this book is available from the
British Library.

ISBN 1 86156 124 5

Printed and bound in the UK by Athenæum Press Ltd,
Gateshead, Tyne & Wear

Contents

List of Contributors

Carolyn Anderson, Department of Speech and Language Therapy, University of Strathclyde

Roberta M. Lees, Department of Speech and Language Therapy, University of Strathclyde

Gilbert MacKay, Department of Special Educational Needs, University of Strathclyde

Margo Mackay, Speech and Language Therapist, Central Scotland Health Care NHS Trust

Elspeth McCartney, Department of Speech and Language Therapy, University of Strathclyde

Susan McCool, Speech and Language Therapist, Renfrewshire and Inverclyde Primary Health Care NHS Trust

Margaret Young, Learning Support Teacher, Stirling Council Education Services

List of Abbreviations

AFASIC	Association for all Speech Impaired Children
BSA	British Stammering Association
CATS	Clinician Attitudes to Stuttering Inventory
CDC	Child Development Centre
CELF	Clinical Evaluation of Language Fundamentals
CLIP	Clinical Language Intervention Programme
CRIL	Criterion Referenced Inventory of Language
CSLT	College of Speech and Language Therapists
CT	Class Teacher
DES	Department of Education
DfE	Department for Education
DfEE	Department for Education and Employment
DoH	Department of Health
EA	Education Authority
ELB	Education and Library Board
ELS	Extended Learning Support
ELST	Extended Learning Support Teacher
EPSEN	Effective Provision for Special Educational Needs
FTE	Full-time Equivalent
HMI	Her Majesty's Inspectorate
HT	Headteacher
IPSEA	Independent Panel for Special Educational Advice
IEP	Individual Education Plan
LDA	Learning Development Aids
LDU	Language Development Unit
LEA	Local Education Authority
MSc	Master of Science
NASEN	National Association for Special Educational Needs
NCC	National Curriculum Council
NHS	National Health Service
Ofsted	Office for Standards in Education
RCSLT	Royal College of Speech and Language Therapists

SEN	Special Educational Needs
SENCO	Special Educational Needs Co-ordinator
SLA	Support for Learning Assistant
SLT	Speech and Language Therapy/Therapist
SOED	Scottish Office Education Department
SOEID	Scottish Office Education and Industry Department
UK	United Kingdom

Introduction: Remit, Limits and Organisation of this Book

ELSPETH McCARTNEY

Remit

This book is about speech and language therapists (SLTs) and teachers working together. It argues that, despite considerable difficulties, there is evidence that good collaborative practice is taking place. It illustrates good practice using a systems framework to structure the discussion.

The ways in which SLTs and teachers and, indeed, any professionals collaborate are strongly influenced by the contexts in which they work. The overriding issue that affects SLTs and teachers and that recurs as a constant theme in the discussion is that these two professions work in separate, large, impressive organisations, each with its own expectations and practices – SLTs in the health service, teachers in education. These organisational systems are equally confident in their approaches to service delivery, but are very different in the ways in which they go about it. Differences between the systems can mean that it is not particularly easy to collaborate. The fact that good collaborative practice does take place is a tribute to the determination and realism of the professionals in the field.

One of the main reasons that collaboration takes place, despite difficulties, is the commitment of both professions to the needs of children, and the professions' congruent aims of helping children communicate. It is evident to practitioners that it is important to help children communicate with their peers in school classes, so that they will 'gain an education', become literate, understand information about the world and develop learning skills, and improve their quality of life by better sharing in the social interactions of childhood. There is also recognition that language teaching is best carried out in rich, real-life contexts, and that these are very well represented in the classroom.

Such factors have provided the trigger for developing collaborative practice. There is now a considerable amount of published work

1

concerning collaboration but this has been somewhat scattered, appearing in journals, professional and government policy statements, research reports and conference presentations. Teachers and SLTs tend to access different literature, which further impedes the development of shared understandings. It seems worthwhile to attempt to collate and structure this material into book form.

The aims of this text therefore are to detail current developments in collaborative practice, to consider these in the context of the systems within which practitioners work and, most importantly, to provide illustrative examples from the field.

The Systems Approach

The book's organisational rationale derives from a systems approach, with one particular model used as the defining framework. This allows discussion of the functions, structures and processes involved in SLT services and education, and the systems environment in which collaboration takes place. The model is derived from the work of Banathy, and is outlined in Chapter 1 and developed in subsequent chapters.

However, the use of a systems approach ties together an essentially practical text. Published examples of collaboration have so far tended to be long on precept but short on example, and this book aims to redress the balance by illustrating the points made wherever possible. Examples are taken from the literature and from practitioners in the field. In particular, the work carried out by students on a postgraduate MSc module concerned with collaborative practice at the University of Strathclyde Department of Speech and Language Therapy has provided a number of examples of current and innovatory practice, reflecting on real issues and small-scale solutions to collaborative problems.

Limits of the Text

The book centres on the particular area of SLTs and teachers collaborating to help children communicate. In this remit, important areas concerning collaboration with other professionals such as physiotherapists and occupational therapists receive little discussion. Discussion of the role of education psychologists is limited, as is consideration of the overall work patterns of teachers and SLTs apart from collaborative practice. Nor is there much consideration of inter-school collaboration, which is well discussed in Gains and Smith (1994), and in other papers in that special-issue journal.

Collaborative work between teachers and SLTs tends, unsurprisingly, to centre around talking and listening aspects of the school curriculum, and these are discussed and exemplified throughout the book. There are other important curricular areas such as maths and science, where children with language and communication difficulties can experience obstacles, predicated on their language problems (Conti-Ramsden et al., 1992). These are areas where SLT–teacher collaboration is developing, and there is also considerable joint work being undertaken in the field of literacy and emergent literacy (McCartney and Wilson, 1994). So far, however, there are not many detailed examples available in these areas. Similarly, there are few examples available from secondary education, although the overall issues around collaboration discussed in the book are relevant to that sector. It is probable that collaborative working in such areas will develop further, and detailed exploration in another context could bear fruit.

The book does not discuss the causes and types of language difficulty in children, nor the variety of approaches used to help children learn language, nor the range of language programmes available. Those interested in introductory information on these topics are referred to Martin and Miller (1996), Daines et al. (1996) and Lees and Urwin (1997); and for detailed discussion of language work within the classroom to Merritt and Culatta (1998), which contains excellent illustrative examples.

Terms and Use of Language

The book is intended to be read cross-professionally, with particular relevance to practitioners in the UK, although the issues raised are pertinent to many other countries. Terms are therefore explained as far as necessary for interprofessional comprehension, but are unapologetically left 'woolly' for large concepts where a general term will suffice. For example, the term 'children with language and communication difficulties' is used throughout the book to encompass a whole range of children, many of whom will have a variety of disabilities and cognitive impairments. It is not intended to imply either that they have specific language disorders or pervasive communication disorders; simply that they have sufficient difficulty in some aspect of understanding or talking to make it difficult to exchange meanings in their social environment, and to access the school curriculum. Throughout the book, examples are given of children with different types of language and communication difficulties, to illustrate aspects of the collaborative process. It is intended and hoped that such difficulties are described in comprehensible terms, but no detailed definitions are given. A glossary of terms and abbreviations is presented at the beginning of the book. System boundaries are also kept at a common sense operational level – there is no detailed analysis of what is meant by terms such as school, education service or SLT service, and such terms may be used fluidly to represent different entities at different times. The abbreviation 'SLT' is used for speech and language therapy or therapist, according to context, and is extended to include equivalent professions outside the UK which properly have different titles, and instances when the title 'speech therapist' would be more historically accurate.

There are particular terminological difficulties in that different parts of the UK use different terms for similar practices. At present England and Wales share one set of legislation: Northern Ireland has another, and Scotland yet another. Legislation in Northern Ireland is closely related to English and Welsh practice, although it is often enacted at a different time and with minor variations. English legal judgments cannot automatically be applied in Northern Ireland, but it is also unlikely that they will be ignored (RCSLT, 1997). The issues that arise in England, Wales and Northern Ireland are therefore fairly similar. Scotland, however, has quite a different set of terms and a separate parliamentary system. Examples of these differences are that purchasers of health services are known as Health Boards in Scotland, as Health Authorities in England and Wales and as Health and Social Services Boards in Northern Ireland. Education Authorities (EAs) fund Scottish schools: Local Education Authorities (LEAs) do so in England and Wales, and Education and Library Boards (ELBs) in Northern Ireland. The highly influential Code of Practice on Special Education Needs, which set up the Special Needs Co-ordinator (SENCO) in England and Wales in 1994, came into full practice in Northern Ireland in 1998, and does not operate in Scotland, although there is a comparable document. Children in England, Wales and Northern Ireland have a statement of special educational needs (SEN) opened to document particular measures needed to help them learn: children in Scotland have a record of SEN to map a similar process. There is a National Curriculum operating in primary schools in England, Wales and Northern Ireland and a 5–14 Curriculum covering similar issues in Scotland. Future devolved parliamentary systems may change the situation still further.

There are important philosophical and legislative differences underpinning such variations in terminology, but these are addressed in this book only where they have particular relevance. If a general point is being made, terms appropriate to most of the UK are used at the risk of some imprecision. Where an example pertains to a particular child or service, however, the locally appropriate term is given.

Organisation of the Book

The book begins by considering the legal and organisational framework in which SLTs and teachers operate in Chapter 1, and the historical developments that have led to this point. There have been substantial alterations to service organisation over time, and this process continues: as the book goes to press, a government action plan arising from a green paper, 'Excellence for All Children', is considering how SLT services to schools outside Scotland should be funded. However, the continued employment of SLTs in the health service and the continued provision of SLT services in school settings are factors that are not expected to change in the near future. The need for consideration of these overall working contexts is met by using a systems approach, and Chapter 1 also outlines this approach.

The fact that collaboration takes place across two major public services creates significant barriers to collaboration, and these are discussed in Chapter 2, using the systems approach outlined in Chapter 1 as the framework for discussion. The chapter argues that functional, structural and systems environment barriers to communication present particular difficulties that must be overcome, but that collaboration at a process level (where decisions are made for individual children) is fairly well developed. There is evidence from the field that all levels of inter-professional barriers are now being recognised and tackled, and that good collaborative practices are evolving at all systems levels. These overall approaches and patterns of collaboration are described in Chapter 3 using the same systems framework.

The book then looks at provision and collaboration in a variety of specialist settings. Chapter 4 considers an example where language units were set up at a rapid rate, and Chapter 5 gives a detailed example of collaboration in an extended learning support facility in a mainstream school.

These two chapters deal with services that are specifically set up for children with language and communication difficulties. Chapter 6 discusses collaboration in mainstream schools, where children with language and communication difficulties can form a very small part of the school population. There are good reasons for educating children in such settings, but the small numbers of children with language and communication difficulties in any one setting can mean that collaboration is difficult to manage, and the chapter outlines current approaches. Chapter 7 considers the difficulties of children who stammer, who do not usually require curriculum adaptations of the type required for children with other language learning difficulties, but whose problems require sensitive handling in school settings.

Chapter 8 considers the role of parents, which is also considered somewhat differently in health and education settings, with implications for parental involvement with children's learning. Chapter 9 considers how services can evaluate the effectiveness of their provision, arguing for a broad systems approach to capture the complexity of what it means to be an 'effective' service.

As stated, examples are used to illustrate good practice, and to provide real-life samples of how problems are being tackled. There is a great deal of good practice to draw upon, and this book can give only a flavour of the complex interaction and collaboration being developed in the field of education. There has been a recent 'sea-change' in practice, and this book captures a particular period of time when a move by teachers and SLTs from independent working to collaborative working is taking place. It is an exciting change, and it is hoped that by documenting some of the relevant issues this book will help to accelerate the process.

Chapter 1
The Legal and
Organisational Framework

ELSPETH McCARTNEY

Introduction

Collaboration between teachers and SLTs takes place across two of the major public-sector organisations in the UK – the health service and the education service. This division in itself creates barriers to collaboration, as discussed in Chapter 2, and the individual perspectives of the two services affect the ways in which teachers and SLTs work to overcome these barriers, as outlined in the rest of the book. That SLTs and teachers work in different systems recurs again and again as a relevant factor in discussing how they collaborate.

However, this division has not always existed. Until the mid-1970s many SLTs were employed in school services, which obviated some of the current problems and caused others. It is helpful to consider historical developments to realise how the relationship between teachers and SLTs has changed over time, and to understand how the present situation has evolved. The first half of this chapter will therefore give an overview of the structural and policy changes that have affected interprofessional collaboration.

A chronological approach is useful for such an account, but other models are needed to understand how services interact. To help this process, a systems model has been adopted throughout much of the text to provide a framework for understanding collaborative practice. The particular model used will be outlined in the second half of this chapter, as an introduction to the discussion in the rest of the book.

The Development of Collaboration – The Historical Picture

Early collaboration

Education provision for children with varieties of language and communication difficulties can be traced back over many years, and some extant

9

services have their origins in the nineteenth century. The establishment of SLT services, however, is more recent and is perhaps best considered as beginning from the formation of the College of Speech Therapists (now the Royal College of Speech and Language Therapists – RCSLT) at the start of 1945. By then, specialist SLT courses had developed to train therapists, and many early SLT students were teachers gaining an additional qualification (Robertson et al., 1995; McCartney, 1996). The links with education were strong.

Postwar developments in SLT service organisation are reviewed by Robertson and colleagues (1995). Around the time that the College of Speech Therapists was formed, the Education Act of 1944 (1945 in Scotland) and the subsequent Ministry of Education's Handicapped Pupils and School Health Service Regulations were passed. These acts governed the education of children with special needs, and adopted a classificatory approach based on a child's handicapping condition. Among other groups, education authorities were required to provide special education for children with 'speech defects'. These were defined as pupils who on account of 'stammering, aphasia or defect of voice or articulation not due to deafness' required special educational 'treatment' (MoE, 1945). These requirements led to a large increase in the number of school clinics with a SLT service, with SLTs employed either by a school medical service or a town education committee. By the early 1950s about 210 SLTs worked in England across some 500 school speech clinics, and another 60 SLTs in Scotland, Wales and Northern Ireland covered 120 clinics. The peripatetic pattern of SLT service delivery was thus formed early, as was the 'extraction' model of therapy out of the classroom – children typically visited a clinic once a week for 'treatment', with parental involvement in therapy. Most of the children had speech difficulties or stammered, but some had cleft palates, cerebral palsy or voice disorders.

The 1960s and 1970s

The numbers of SLTs continued to grow throughout the 1960s, and parallel services developed in hospital and health service settings, which included work with adult clients. A government committee of inquiry into the SLT profession was set up in 1969 and reported in 1972 (Quirk, 1972). It recommended a unified organisation for the whole of the SLT profession, with all SLTs to be based in the field of health. This recommendation was implemented from 1974 as part of an overall National Health Service reorganisation in which area health authorities/boards were set up. SLTs were thus all employed in the health service, and integrated into coherent teams serving the needs of the whole adult and child population in any geographical area. SLT specialisms developed, and services were supplied to schools and school clinics. The somewhat anomalous position, which still exists, was thus established whereby many SLTs were employed by health services but spent much of their working life in schools.

Until the start of the 1970s, health services had also looked after children who had special educational needs of such severity that they were deemed 'ineducable'. At that point, however, the rights of all children to education were recognised, and all children were brought into school settings for at least the statutory school years (Wedell, 1993). Throughout the 1970s special schools and special provision remained classified principally according to children's category of disability, although there was a move to try to include many children in mainstream schools.

The 1980s and 1990s

SLTs

Three major policy developments during the 1980s and 1990s had an impact on collaborative practice between SLTs and teachers. One was in the health service and two in education. SLTs, employed by the health service, were affected by the extensive changes following the publication and implementation of the government paper 'Working for Patients' (DoH, 1989). This introduced a split between 'purchasers' of health services, which now became the role of health authorities/ boards and of some general practitioners; and 'providers' of services, which were set up as NHS trusts, employing healthcare staff, including SLTs. This created a new internal market, where trusts 'sold' services to commissioning purchasers. In the case of SLT services these changes often meant fragmentation, as the new trusts tended to be smaller than the former area-wide services, and tended to deal with specific client groups; adult and children's services were frequently separated. The introduction of a market also meant that costs and charges tended to become a focus of service organisation, which caused, and still causes, particular difficulties in organising collaboration, as will be discussed.

Teachers

Teachers in schools in the meantime were affected by the two interacting issues of a reconceptualisation of the special educational needs of children, and the introduction of nationwide approaches to the school curriculum.

The important reconceptualisation of children's special educational needs involved moving away from categorising children according to handicapping conditions. These came to be seen as a limiting factor that tended to place too much emphasis on a child's 'deficit' and not enough on the actions needed to help children learn. Following publication of the influential Warnock report in 1978, education acts in the early 1980s concentrated on these issues. The acts abolished the categories of 'handicap' and replaced them with the term 'learning difficulties'. This related to children who were having significantly greater difficulty in learning than most children of their age, or who had a disability that hindered their use of the education facilities generally provided by the local authority. Specific provision was to be made for them, in addition to, or different from, that offered to other children. Inclusion of the child in mainstream school settings was seen to be the 'default' condition for education provision, to be implemented wherever possible. Procedures were set up to make a detailed account of the child's needs and the actions to be taken to meet those needs, in the form of a statement or record of special educational needs.

However, it was never intended that all children with special needs would go through the full procedures for opening a statement or record. Indeed, it was intended that only about 2% of children would require a statutory assessment of needs. Another and much larger group of children, perhaps another 18%, would at some time require special help in school, which could be dealt with by action within a school and by good educational practices to help the child to learn. Procedures to refine the process of identifying and meeting children's special needs were implemented in England and Wales in 1994 (and in Northern Ireland in 1998) with the publication of a code of practice on the identification and assessment of special educational needs (DfE, 1994). This was a mandatory statement that clarified roles and responsibilities, the stages for action and the time limits within which action should be taken. It identified stopping-off points, which meant that learning needs that could be dealt with at school level could be described and acted on efficiently.

The code of practice stressed school and SLT partnership: in presenting the code in the House of Lords Baroness Blatch commented:

> We have also sought to improve the guidance on speech and language therapy. Throughout, the code lays particular emphasis on partnership. Nowhere is such partnership more important than in meeting the needs of children with speech and language difficulties (Hansard, 1994: 1414).

Unfortunately, issues around funding SLT input were not dealt with in the code, which therefore maintained an area of difficulty which still pertains.

In the same year a cognate good practice document was published in Scotland, entitled 'Effective Provision for Special Education Needs' (the 'EPSEN document' – SOEID, 1994). This offered advice and guidance similar to the code of practice in relation to recording children's special needs, but does not have mandatory status.

Although procedures for opening a statement or record of special education needs are firmly set in an education context, there was (and is) a place for SLT input in the form of advice, and for SLT inclusion in the annual review of the statement or record for children for whom SLT provision has been made. SLT advice aims to be clear enough to give other professionals and parents an understanding of the child's educational needs. A summary of therapy required to help the child towards achieving independence and to develop educationally, and of the facilities and resources recommended to achieve these aims, is to be given (RCSLT, 1996: 222-3).

The emphasis on identifying special needs is therefore firmly on the actions that relevant professionals are to carry out in the school system to adapt the learning environment to meet a child's needs, rather than on a child's inherent difficulties. However, the code of practice reintroduced some specific points relating to disabilities, including speech and language difficulties. This focus on special learning needs was less wholeheartedly adopted in health services, where an emphasis on the 'medical' model of identifying areas of deficit in a child and attempting to remediate these remained common. Both approaches have merits in specific contexts, but an unfortunate divergence of approach between SLTs in the health service and teachers in education was suggested. This became a potential barrier to collaborative work, as the language and expectations of teachers and SLTs grew apart.

The second major education policy initiative to affect collaboration was the adoption of national curricula, which laid down frameworks for work to be carried out by all children in school, and for ways of assessing children's attainments (DES, 1989; SOED, 1991/93). There were some differences in the curricula operating in different parts of the UK: policy on national curricula once more assumed mandatory status in England, Wales and Northern Ireland, but remained at the level of strong advice and guidance in Scotland. Both curricula, however, stress the importance to primary school children of talking and listening to help them learn. There were instances where the curriculum could be 'disapplied' for children with special educational needs (Emblem and Conti-Ramsden, 1990), but, overall, educationists accepted the principle of attempting to include all children in the curriculum wherever possible, and of finding ways of differentiating within the curriculum framework to meet children's needs (DES, 1989; SOEID, 1994: 40).

The adoption of a national curricular approach to speaking and listening had a great impact on collaborative work between teachers and SLTs. There are some interprofessional difficulties, as discussed in the next chapter, created by the very fact of having a curriculum, and the UK versions did not necessarily use approaches familiar to SLTs. However, the overriding impact of having communication on the list of issues to be addressed in school provided a significant impetus for collaboration. It provided a framework for discussing language, and new ways of considering children with language and communication difficulties. As the effect of the curriculum became apparent, Peacey (1992) noted:

> This heightened concern about language in schools means that the SLT's work has changed for ever. If children with speech and language difficulties are to have the curriculum that is their legal entitlement, teachers and SLTs have to collaborate (p. 11).

Funding for SLT

Such policy initiatives did not, however, deal with a major barrier to collaboration which had arisen by the end of the 1980s. This concerned funding for SLT services. Since SLTs were based in health services, the question of who would fund their services in education settings had become a difficult issue. Many children were receiving statements of special educational need that stipulated that SLT services were needed, and at times how much SLT input should be given. However, education authorities making such statements did not employ SLTs, and could not always command sufficient input from health service provision to fulfil these obligations. Parents were upset and confused when this happened, and several legal actions were raised. In 1989 an individual case was heard in the High Court (Regina v. Lancashire County Council 1989) which dealt with the matter. The 'Lancashire judgment', as it became known, ruled that, for most children with statements of special educational needs listing SLT input, such input was an education provision, and should therefore be included in the appropriate education section of the statement. The judge, Lord Justice Balcombe, noted:

> To teach an adult who has lost his larynx because of cancer might well be considered as treatment rather than education. But to teach a child who has never been able to communicate by language, whether because of some chromosomal disorder ... or because of some social cause (e.g. because his parents are themselves unable to speak, and thus he cannot learn by example as normally happens) seems to us just as much educational provision as to teach a child to communicate in writing (AFASIC, 1993: 1).

However, this judgment applied to most children, not all. This meant that in individual cases SLT input could be seen as either a special educational provision, as in the Lancashire judgment instances, or non-educational. Where it was seen as a special educational provision the child's LEA could look, in the first instance, to health services to provide therapy. However, should the health services be unable to do so, it remained the education authority's duty to secure the provision of SLT. No extra funds were given for this, and it was difficult to see how education authorities could secure such provision.

In other instances, SLT provision could be seen as non-educational, in which case education authorities had no responsibility to provide it. No clear distinction between SLT as a non-educational provision and SLT as educational provision was made, and the lack of clarity persisted in the code of practice which repeated the confusing advice without guidance as to what differentiating factors might be (Miller, 1994). This situation was not very helpful to collaborative practice, as the supply of SLT services to children with special needs remained insecure.

A policy review forum had been held by the SLT profession to debate this issue in advance of the publication of the code (CSLT, 1993a), where SLTs expressed concern lest access to SLT services for school children should only be built around statementing/recording procedures which would apply to only a minority of children. Such concerns remained, and the profession's commitment to the principle that access to SLT services should be seen as essential across the whole spectrum of individual needs and not as a priority for pupils with statements or records of need was restated in principles and guidelines published four years later (RCSLT, 1997: 3).

The 1993 forum also noted that demand for SLT services had increased rapidly, with no corresponding supply of staff. Indeed, the number of SLTs employed in the UK by the late 1990s remained small in relation to the number of teachers. (A comparison in Scotland for 1996 where all teachers in local authority schools and most teachers in independent schools are registered, suggests a ball park figure of about 100 times more registered teachers than SLTs in practice. Similar figures probably pertain in other parts of the UK, and in this context management of demand will no doubt remain an issue for some time to come.)

The funding of SLT provision in schools in Scotland had been, and remains, somewhat different to that in the rest of the UK. The Secretary of State for Scotland was faced with similar issues around funding, and similar parental disquiet, and acted decisively to deal with the problem. In 1991 he gave Scottish education authorities funds to purchase SLT services for those children with a record of needs where SLT input was considered to be a special educational need. Education authorities arranged contracts through health boards, which contracted with trusts to supply SLT services. This situation in itself raised difficulties (which will be referred to again in Chapter 2) and still applied to only the small number of children who had specific advice about SLT provision in their record of special educational needs. However, the additional money defused much of the problem in Scotland and provided one creative alternative to the problems of securing funding.

The current situation

As the 1990s end, the situation whereby SLTs remain in the health service but offer services in education settings seems likely to continue, more particularly in light of the SLT profession's decision to join the Council for Professions Supplementary to Medicine (Montgomery, 1998). Only one or two education authorities in the UK (for example, Newham and Dyfed) have chosen to set up, fund, employ and manage their own SLT service. The educational setting for many children with language and communication difficulties seems likely to be the mainstream school, both for reasons of social equity and to provide the rich environment in which children's education can best take place. Collaboration between teachers and SLTs is developing rapidly, although the issue of funding for SLT services in education settings, for children with records or statements of special educational needs and for those without, remains problematic. A government green paper for England and Wales (and later Northern Ireland) entitled 'Excellence for all Children' (DfEE, 1997) devoted four paragraphs to the provision of speech and language therapy in schools (pp. 72, 73). It noted the need for collaboration between school and SLT services to be improved as a key to raising the educational potential of children with language and communication difficulties. The green paper recognised the difficulties posed by lack of clarity over funding, and suggested that either the Scottish model be used for children with statements, or that joint responsibility between education and health authorities for funding and managing SLT services for all children be adopted, which would allow coordination throughout schools and with pre-school services.

Following consultation, however, no clear decision has been made. Instead, a working group has been established to undertake a 'scoping study' to review the whole area (DfEE 1998). It is suggested that this study might include further research into the effectiveness of SLT for children with SEN; develop pilot projects on innovative provision; develop principles for the effective planning and delivery of SLT and offer practical guidance for parents on SLT services and parents' role in supporting therapy (p. 20). Views are sought on the terms in which SLT provision should be described (DfEE 1999).

It therefore appears that the issue of SLT work in schools remains on the political agenda. Debate will take place within a new holistic approach to collaboration which is developing across legislation for health, education and social services in England (DfEE 1998, DoH 1998, McCartney 1999) and which sets up a new 'duty of partnership' amongst services. This new function is intended to ease barriers to joint working across services, and to produce a 'seamless service' for clients. Details of how SLT services are to be organised in school will be worked out within this context, which should help to facilitate purposeful collaborative practice.

A Systems Model

Along with curriculum approaches in education and purchaser contracts in health has come a general emphasis on demonstrating effectiveness in public services and new approaches to service evaluation. The ways in which education and health services have attempted to measure effectiveness differ quite markedly, as will be discussed in Chapter 9. However, approaches to evaluating services are all ultimately concerned with gaining a holistic picture of services and their effects on children's lives, and flexible, interactive and responsive approaches are needed which are none the less systematic. The approach adopted in this book is that described by McCartney et al. (1998) based on a systems approach proposed by Hungarian social scientist Béla Banathy (1973, 1992, 1996; and see also MacKay et al., 1993, 1995).

Banathy's model is useful because of its firm location in education settings, but with applications also to health services. He uses helpful visual imagery, considering 'bird's-eye', 'moving-picture' and 'still-picture' as images for the three main 'models' of his system. An outline of his approach is given here to explain the starting point and main features of the approach. The components of Banathy's three-part model will be described (Banathy, 1992), which move from a general understanding of any system to a detailed examination of its operation, and then the four-part adaptation found useful by McCartney et al. (1998) will be discussed.

Banathy's three-level model

1 The 'bird's-eye model': 'systems-environment'

The systems-environment model allows us to describe a system such as a school, SLT service or other form of provision in the context of its community and of the larger society. Banathy (1992, 1996) sees this model as a lens through which to have a bird's-eye view of the landscape in which the system is sited. The systems-environment model examines how the system being studied, and the individuals and other systems with which it comes into contact, relate, interact and are interdependent. This outlook encourages questions about how adequately the service being studied responds to the context in which it is set, and conversely about how responsive that context is to the service on offer. In the case of an SLT service or school there are many layers of social influence, but the relation between the service and the local health purchaser and education authority, and the relationship between the service and the families of its clients, are areas of inquiry where the systems-environment outlook is particularly appropriate.

2 The 'moving-picture model': 'process'

This model helps to direct attention to what a system does across a period of time. It concerns changes in the system, but can also focus on children as learners and the processes of children's engagement with the system to achieve their learning objectives.

Typically, it is concerned with:

- input to the system, including the child's learning needs on enrolment in a school or referral to an SLT service and the system's ways of conceptualising and identifying these
- operations through which children undergo change and learn, such as a classroom or therapy programme, and the adjustments made to these operations to optimise learning
- output processes by which learning is measured and children eventually move on from the system being studied, for example by transferring to another school or being discharged from a therapy service; and feedback and adjustment concerned with interpreting and developing the system.

The process approach may be used, simply, to chart a child's contact with a service, along the path of referral, admission, provision, review and, eventually, transfer (although this list could be extended). Such charting can also be useful for generating questions about the whole system, or about parts of it, and may yield guidance on the more effective operation of the system. The overall aim is to achieve this by an understanding of the system as an active entity, hence the 'moving-picture' analogy.

3 The 'still-picture model': 'functions/structures'

Banathy's 'functions/structures model' is a development of the 'general still-picture model' of schooling described in Banathy (1973), which is based on the principle that systems exist for the purpose of achieving goals. It is therefore concerned with features of a system, such as its goals (including education goals), the functions it carries out to meet these goals (such as organising the learning environment), and the components required to carry out these functions (such as subsystems to do with teaching and administration). The functions/structure model takes metaphorical snapshots of these aspects, which act as points of reference against which to examine past and future practice.

In this model, analysis of goals leads to the identification of functions that the system has to carry out in order to achieve its goals. Goals would often include broad social aims to do with individuals realising their full potential, and developing the community as a learning society. These refine down to functions such as providing access to learning experiences, providing resources, making arrangements and monitoring these functions.

Investigation of the functions of a service will reveal who and what are required to carry out these functions. This is likely to lead, first, to the specification of a set of subsystems such as governance, school administration and instruction, in a school context (Banathy, 1992: 89). Banathy's 'components' are the substance of these subsystems, and include human and material resources. The components of the 'instruction' subsystem include children, teachers, classrooms, books and other materials, interconnected by a set of relationships. The components of the 'therapy' subsystem could also be said to include children, SLTs, therapy settings and materials, and the relationships between them. Similarly, school and SLT services, administration and the other subsystems have their own sets of patterned relationships.

In this framework, system boundaries exist between schools and SLT services, and each will have its own set of subsystems. Banathy considers that the more that subsystems are segregated in any system, the more likely is the degeneration of the system as a whole. Consequently, the integration of subsystems by communication among them has a special place in enabling the system to meet its goals. In considering collaborative approaches, the relationships between subsystems in the two overarching 'suprasystems' of health and education services will also be important.

Beyond the 'functions/structures model'

Research into small-scale education evaluation has led to development of the third of Banathy's components, the 'functions/structures' model. Banathy regards goals, functions and components as being bound together in a single model, the 'still-picture', which describes how systems are at a given moment. However, in his later writing, Banathy (1992, 1996) draws more attention to the relational arrangements within and among components, by calling them 'structures', and by changing the name of the 'still-picture model' to the 'functions/structure model'.

Banathy argues that a consideration of functions is a logically necessary first step in systems evaluation, and counsels against a 'celebration' of organisational structure (Banathy, 1992: 92). He maintains the centrality of function in his functions/structures model. However, when considering collaborative practice many organisational features are already set up when professionals begin to collaborate, especially in large systems such as education and health services. For these reasons, MacKay et al. (1993, 1995) and McCartney et al. (1998) considered it helpful to discuss 'structures' as a discrete category, in order to provide a clearer context in which to ask certain questions. This is partly because of discontent with Banathy's assertion that: 'the goal – functions – component sequence is obligatory' (Banathy, 1973: 23).

This sequence may be ideal, but it cannot be obligatory, for such an assertion is based on the assumption that services undergo a rational process of planning and implementation from a fresh start. In practice, all sorts of 'components', and the structures that link them, are likely to exist as robust features of the environment in which collaboration takes place. For collaborating professions these prior categories will affect the actions that can be taken. Collaborating colleagues are not designing systems, but are trying to operate within existing parameters. However sensible it may be to consider the goals and functions of an organisation before setting up the structures with which it is to run, SLTs and teachers will not usually have much option about structural matters, but will be trying to work in the given organisational arrangements.

For these reasons, it is useful to re-examine the dimension that describes how the goals of a service are achieved. This dimension can be considered to have two major poles: the functions, or the means by which goals are achieved; and the structures, which concern the internal organisation of these functions, and the relationships among and between them. The following examples may help. The function of increasing SLTs' and teachers' understanding of collaborative working may be effected by structures such as joint working parties and in-service programmes. The function of parental empowerment may be effected by attention to the development of structures such as parents' groups and explicit lines of communication.

MacKay et al. (1993, 1995) and McCartney et al. (1998) have therefore adapted Banathy's models and used the four dimensions of functions, structures, process and systems-environment for guidance in the formulation of questions about small-scale education-influenced organisations, and in the development of instruments to answer them. These dimensions have proved useful in giving a framework to discuss the large and diverse amount of detail available in considering collaboration, and in tracing a path through complexity. These four dimensions will be used in this book. The following descriptions of the issues that appear relevant under these headings should help to explain the book's organisational framework.

The functions model

This model for understanding a system is concerned with describing the goals of the system, and the functions it carries out to meet these goals. Perhaps the first step is to consider what the service intends to provide, and how it intends to provide. This is usually available from analysis of policy statements, and the principles to which a service commits. In the context of collaboration, there are education, health service and professional policy statements at all levels which document what a service is trying to achieve; there has been extensive development of such documentation in recent years. Policies would probably contain information on the service's overall aims for the children who access it, and ideally the aims of collaborative practice would also be mentioned. Measures of how well an individual service was fulfilling its functions could be gained from interviews with relevant individuals, audit and inspection measures and consideration of its relationship with its community environment. Aggregate measures of children's progress, obtained on an individual basis at the process level, could also be used to evaluate functional effectiveness.

There are major differences in the ways in which health and education services select the children who will access services, and how they group and classify children and children's language learning difficulties. SLTs and teachers may have different models of how professionals work together, and may know little about one another's working life. These areas will be explored in the next two chapters, first in Chapter 2 as barriers that can impede collaboration, and then in Chapter 3 with examples of how such barriers might be overcome.

The structures model

The structures model as employed here is used to describe the decision-making procedures and the formalised ways in which parts of a service relate to other parts, including the structured ways in which opinion is sought by the service. It also deals with relatively consistent aspects of the context, such as the school year and timetable, and relatively permanent features of organisation such as how children are grouped in classes and how SLT services are managed. As with functions, structures can also be gauged by analysis of formal documentation (such as therapy mission statements and school plans) and by discussion with policy-makers and staff, and evaluated in the ways that functions can. It is probably easier to think of structures in an education setting, but SLTs are employed in NHS trusts, which have their own line-management structures and reporting and record-keeping structures.

Differences that arise are discussed as barriers in Chapter 2 and revisited when discussing patterns of collaboration in Chapter 3. These concern the timing and location of service delivery, management structures and curriculum structures.

The process model

A process model focuses inquiry on how the system behaves. In the context of collaborative practice it can be used to understand how that service affects the lives of the people within it; children, families, professionals and others.

The process model used is based on the assumption that the contact of every child with a service follows a series of events. The start of this series is the child's referral or admission to the service; events continue through the learning experiences provided for the child with the end-point as the completion of transition to new education provision or discharge from the SLT service, and perhaps further to aspects of the child's future career. Banathy (1992) offers useful guidance on the development of a process model. It should note how a service receives referrals, and how it assesses the needs of the children referred. It should then show how this information is used in the life of the service. Taking stock of the total picture presented by the process model allows judgements to be made on the adequacy of service functioning. Evaluation can involve an analysis of how an individual child makes progress with their individual goals, and the aggregate of such measures can feed back into the function model to see how a whole service is performing.

In connection with collaboration in schools, the issues identified for discussion in Chapters 2 and 3 are decisions around whether or not to set up a statement or record of special educational needs, and the construction of an individual education plan for a child.

Systems-environment model

This model shows how a system fits the context of its community and the larger society. It deals with identifying concepts and principles that govern relationships and interactions among the individuals and agencies who constitute the wider context. The model may also be used in the opposite way to examine the responsiveness of the environment to the service. Since the goals of a service may be different from the space made for it in the environment in which it is to operate, it is helpful to investigate the meaning that the service has in the minds of its users and potential users. In the context of teacher and SLT collaboration, one of the most important perspectives is that of children's families, and this will receive considerable attention in this book, both in the next two chapters and in Chapter 8. Other relevant components of the systems environment might include voluntary groups and charities concerned with the well-being of children with language and communication difficulties. Whereas the process, functions and structures models are particularly appropriate for examining the perceptions of the providers of a service, the systems-environment model illuminates the response of its users. (see Summary on p.23.)

The holistic picture

Using systems approaches to record the perspectives of a system's providers and users provides a wealth of information offering different insights into many of the same issues. Individual outlooks can be compared, which can aid the conceptualisation of services as three-dimensional living systems, embedded in fuller networks, and interacting in various dimensions. The use of the systems analysis approach also provides a framework that helps to organise information, and to

Summary of the systems model	
Functions *The goals of the system*	**Structures** *Formal decision-making mechanisms*
Relevant to collaboration are: prioritisation of children differentiation versus deficit models of practice models of interprofessional working social interaction	**Relevant to collaboration are:** timing and location of service delivery management structures curriculum structures
Process *How a system behaves*	**Systems environment** *How a system fits into its community*
Relevant to collaboration are: statements or records of SENs individual education plans	**Relevant to collaboration are:** social expectations voluntary organisations parents and families

draw a purposeful path through complexity. Pointers for service development can emerge, and the iterative nature of the analysis means that change over time can be tracked.

However, information can cross model boundaries; for example, knowing about children's attainment of their individual language goals not only helps monitor process but also helps in the consideration of functions, structures and the systems environment. A systems model provides a flexible and sensitive way of gathering information, which retains a proper emphasis on complexity and different professional perspectives, but which allows discussion of 'good' service provision from the point of view of all participants and users. It will be used as an organising framework throughout much of the book.

Chapter 2
Barriers to Collaboration

ELSPETH McCARTNEY

Introduction

As the last chapter outlined, the current outcome of a set of legal and organisational decisions is that SLT services and schools operate in two separate public-sector divisions: schools within education and SLTs within health. In these major organisations they provide different kinds of services, and operate in different social systems and with major differences in philosophy and organisation. Schools within education services have their own strong context and expectations: SLTs within health services have a different but equally strong context and assumptions about service delivery. It is important to discuss these differences, and to bring them into the open, so that problems, issues and barriers to collaboration that arise from organisational differences can be explained.

Barriers to Collaboration

Collaboration is self-evidently considered to be a 'good thing', and the ways in which it can benefit children are discussed in the next chapter. There is therefore considerable encouragement at policy and legislative level for SLTs and teachers to collaborate. Despite this, there are serious obstacles to collaboration. Dessent (1996) crystallises the general problems in collaboration as discussed by a variety of authors into a useful list, which summarises just how hard it can be to implement collaboration. His list of difficulties (see page 25) provides a useful starting point for discussion.

Almost all of these factors apply to relationships between SLTs and teachers, and suggest that the barriers to collaborative working are considerable. A similar review of issues concerning collaboration brings

Davie (1993) to worry that, despite wide professional recognition of the value of collaborative approaches:

> the prevailing system is heavily loaded against multi-professional co-operation. If one were to attempt – with all the insights derived from research and common experience – to establish a process designed to keep the professionals apart, it would be difficult to conceive of any improvement on what we currently have (p. 140).

Obstacles to collaboration – Dessent's example

Organisational/structural
- Different services administered by different agencies
- Large, complex agencies with multiple subsystems
- Lack of 'co-terminosity' in agency boundaries

Professional
- Separate training and conceptual background
- Different vocabulary relating to 'need' (medical/education)
- Different pay, conditions and status
- Interprofessional rivalry (power and decision making)
- Loyalty to own agency/service

Legislation
- One agency has principal 'ownership'
- Legislation 'overload'
- Discrete statutory responsibilities
- Poor transferability and cross-referencing of legislation

Resources
- Funding channelled to separate committees and agencies
- Limited 'corporate' budgets
- Resource constraints
- Lack of clarity about budget responsibilities
- Conflicting policy priorities
- Partnership work is time-consuming and expensive

Political/attitudinal
- Lack of political/managerial commitment to inter-agency cooperation
- Lack of officer faith in effectiveness of inter-agency cooperation

Pressures
- 'Innovation overload'
- Agencies dominated by internal priorities
- Restructurings

Dessent (1996)

This is not a happy picture, and teachers and SLTs are working together faced by a background of difficulties before they begin. This chapter explores these difficulties in detail, with particular examples relating to each profession's perspectives. Subsequent chapters give examples of how such barriers are being overcome, but it is necessary first to reflect on the obstacles put in place so that the context of collaboration can be understood.

The Systems Approach

In discussing these issues, the systems approach outlined in the previous chapter will be used as a framework to specify and amplify Dessent's approach and to incorporate helpful examples (Banathy, 1992, 1996). Schools and SLT services will be described, as will the education and health services in which they are embedded, although not all services will have identical characteristics. Since health and education are UK-wide public services subject to national legislation, there is probably sufficient commonality to justify this approach. Banathy explored his model in relation to schools, but also gave examples from healthcare systems.

The adaptation of Banathy's 1992 model outlined in the previous chapter offers four headings within which to consider the differences between schools and SLT services: the functional level, the structural level, the process level and the systems-environment level. These will be considered in turn, with consideration of barriers to collaboration operating at these levels, and examples from the literature of the difficulties that can arise. The four models interconnect, and influence one another, and so issues raised under one model will affect other parts of the organisations (McCartney et al., 1998), but the systems approach allows a flexible framework in which to structure discussion.

Functional Barriers

Functions are considered in the adapted model to be the means by which goals are set and achieved. Schools and SLTs carry out rather different functions. Two major areas of functional difference can be identified for comment: notions of who the service is provided for (all children for education versus targeted children for health, leading to pathology or deficit models of intervention); and different models of interprofessional interaction, including social interaction.

All children versus targeted children

One fundamental difference between health and education services is discussed in McCartney and van der Gaag (1996). They note that education is an allocating service – children receive a fixed number of years in school irrespective of their individual circumstances, and indeed irrespective of how they personally perceive the benefits of schooling. The health service is a commissioning service, where intervention is offered only to targeted children and when a specific need arises: 'unnecessary' intervention in the wider health context is seen as an assault. The health service is also increasingly a prioritising service (RCSLT, 1996: 71 et seq.), where the needs of an individual are balanced against the competing needs of another individual for the same service. To that extent the health service is a rationing service, where decisions about resource allocation are based on both evidence of effectiveness and the overall resources needed to attain predicted results.

Health services have had to consider resource allocation at a fundamental level, from examining what aspects of impairment will even be considered as a health service responsibility (such as aspects of care of the elderly) to managing waiting lists and reducing the cost of services. Health service policies encourage selection of appropriate clients to receive services and assume that they can be differentiated from the normal population – the notion of 'caseness'. There are particular problems in deciding which children with language and communication difficulties should count as 'cases', particularly when many such difficulties can be thought of as lying on the continuum of language ability and not diverging from it (Dale and Cole, 1991; Leonard, 1991).

'Cases' in the health service are further prioritised according to the urgency with which they are to receive a particular service. SLTs have been involved in this process, and as providers of services have been encouraged to outline their service allocation context and principles (DoH, 1989, 1992). Therapists have become increasingly involved in prioritising, monitoring and evaluating their service (Meikle, 1996) and the amount of provision and levels of service offered have been keenly debated. An aim is to achieve equal access to the limited resources available.

These concepts are less fundamental in education, where there is a notion of some equal amount of school provision and resource, and access to an agreed curriculum to be provided for each school-age child. Society has made a decision based on notions of economic and social good that all young children will spend an allocated amount of time in the school setting – in the UK between the ages of 5 and 16 years. This allocation is designed to offer general education benefits, and is associated with notions of citizenship, quality of life and personal opportunity, along with general gains to society arising from the aggregate influence of the education process. The allocation of education to children has come to be seen as a right, and is one that for the past two decades at least has been offered to all children, including those with special needs. A great deal of legal and educational practice has grown up around the allocation and philosophy of schooling and it is in this rich context that schools operate.

Variation in access to, and amount of, education occurs outside the statutory childhood school years, but children are encouraged to stay in education and training after the legal school leaving age. Indeed the notion of a 'lifetime of learning' and continuing professional development is current, where adults continue to use education services, although not usually school services, throughout their lives. There is no notion of an excess of education – learning, as a product of education, is rather seen as a universal good.

Some prioritisation parallels with health services can be found in relation to the issue of allocating additional support to children with special educational needs, but debates around who will receive basic services have not been necessary in education, and indeed are viewed with distaste by many teachers. The background assumption of school staff about children's rights to service may mean that they find the prioritising processes within the NHS model unacceptable. An SLT service that, in education terms, cannot deliver intervention to pupils may be seen as ineffective.

A related barrier to collaborative work can arise when children are selected for help by one service but not the other. A well-documented instance provides an example:

Prioritisation problems – an example

Shaw and colleagues in an SLT service (Shaw et al., 1996; AFASIC, 1997; Luscombe, personal communication, 1998) were awarded additional funding to develop a school-based SLT service for children with special educational needs attending local mainstream schools. They devised a carefully planned approach to offering SLT services for children with special needs in mainstream schools. They carried out a needs assessment, analysed the appropriate mode and frequency of SLT provision, and adopted collaborative working practices. However, SLT resources meant that it would not be possible to fully meet the needs of all children throughout the school year. It was decided with the agreement of the LEA and health authority purchasers to offer schools in half of the local geographical clusters SLT input every other half-term, so that every child would receive their identified level of input in school on a half-termly rotation (Shaw et al., 1996: 331).

Within the first two terms of introducing such a service the number of referrals made it clear that, in the absence of new resources, service levels could not be maintained in the following year. Prioritisation measures were then set up (jointly with colleagues in physiotherapy and occupational therapy) that allocated children to categories of higher or lower priority according to clinical needs for SLT services, regardless of a statement of special education need. Clinical prioritisation factors were a mix of needs factors (age, with young children receiving priority; severity of impairment; need for special aids/equipment) and factors concerning the potential benefits of intervention (related to communication levels compared with overall levels of functioning; stability of the child's condition and so on). This meant that services were withdrawn over time from low-priority groups, and targeted at those who needed them most and had the greatest potential to benefit. However, rising referral rates meant that, despite some staff increases, further prioritisation had to be carried out and a reduction of provision across the service took place, so that each child received 50% of what they required (Luscombe and Shaw, 1996).

Such carefully planned prioritisation of service provision is exemplary practice in health service terms, but in some cases caused distress to parents and the SLTs involved (Luscombe and Shaw, 1996: 9). It also meant that some children with a statement of SENs that specified SLT input were not offered such input. A 6-year-old girl with cerebral palsy was assessed as requiring weekly SLT input to provide direct therapy and advise school staff as appropriate. She received only half the recommended input, i.e. SLT every other week. Her parents took the issue ultimately to the High Court, where the LEA argued that it was relieved of its obligation to fulfil the statement because the local health authority had failed to provide appropriate resources. In the judicial review the judge ruled that: 'the health authority and trust had been "impeccable" in the prioritising of the service and the principle of achieving equity within the available resources' (Luscombe and Shaw, 1996: 9). However, the judge further ruled that the LEA had to make special educational provision for children in accordance with their statements of special educational needs. Part 3 of a child's statement lists the educational provision to be offered, and when SLT input appeared in that section LEAs had a duty to provide it. There was no 'let-out' for the LEA because sufficient resources were not forthcoming from the local health authority.

This is an unhappy example in that good collaborative practice ran into difficulties because of an imbalance between need and resources. The differences between an allocating service, where children have a right to special input, and a prioritising service, where children's needs compete, are clearly shown. This illustrates a fundamental difference between health and education services, which will continue to have a profound effect on collaborative practice across the two services for the foreseeable future.

Educational provision versus 'deficit' models of practice

Schools are concerned with adapting and structuring children's learning experiences so that they can gain optimal benefit from their schooling. Children with special needs require educators to carry out particular actions in an education setting to help them access the curriculum, and these are specified in records or statements of special educational needs, where these exist, and in Individual Education Plans (IEPs). The philosophical basis for considering education in this way can be traced back at least 20 years to the work of the Warnock Committee (DES, 1978), which construed special educational needs as:

not caused solely by deficiencies *within* the child. They result from interaction between the strengths and weaknesses of the child and the resources and deficiencies in the environment. SENs occur in a continuum of degree of severity, and so it is not meaningful to attempt to draw a hard and fast line between the 'handicapped' and the 'non-handicapped' (Wedell, 1993: 2).

This has resulted in schools quite properly looking to what they need to do to enable children to benefit from the curriculum. The key notion is 'differentiation' – defined by Visser (1993) as:

'the process whereby teachers meet the need for progress through the curriculum by selecting appropriate teaching methods to match an individual child's learning strategies, within a group situation' (p. 15).

Education services have therefore concentrated on devising good teaching methods to help foster children's abilities, rather than on trying to 'cure' a disability. Key strategies suggesting how differentiation can be accomplished are outlined in SOED (1993: 28).

Differentiation – examples of key strategies

Individualisation – the specification of particular programmes for individual children whose curriculum requirements call for a judicious selection and arrangement of curricular elements to be taught in particular settings and in deliberate ways. This is used to form the basis of the Individual Education Plan (IEP).

Adaptation – where the curriculum learning outcomes, strands and attainment targets are adapted to meet the specified needs of some pupils, while the broader features of the curriculum remain in place. For example, talking and listening curriculum areas could be adapted to take account of signing or the use of word processors.

Enhancement – which implies introducing or supplementing curriculum aspects that have previously been narrowed or neglected to increase the breadth or depth of children's knowledge. Such work is often carried out by teachers to compensate for children's inexperience.

Elaboration – where the curriculum is developed by producing additional learning outcomes, strands or attainment targets for a child or children which are not otherwise part of a national curriculum. An example would be a specific language programme for children with language disorders.

SOED (1993)

The whole school is involved in setting appropriate special educational policies and encouraging a helpful learning environment. Such approaches do not ignore children's disabilities, and indeed examples of how differentiation might work in practice often refer to disabling conditions. However, the emphasis is less on the child and his or her disabilities as on the appropriate actions to be taken by a school to help a child learn.

SLTs have traditionally adopted a more 'pathological' model, where they assess a child, decide on whether or not there is a problem and outline areas of particular strengths and difficulties. They then plan intervention, often on an individual basis, carry it out and reassess to measure progress. The cycle is perhaps repeated. Such an 'episode of care' once again reflects common health service practices, deriving ultimately from medical models of disability. Indeed, in a strong version of this model, if the child proves not to have sufficient difficulty (and so is not deemed to have 'case' status) intervention is not offered. But in so far as such procedures tend to locate difficulties in the child, rather than in the child's learning environment, and try to deal with them directly, they differ from many current education planning procedures.

Such differences in starting points can cause problems for collaborative work. However, accommodations can be made. Current educational thinking accepts that both the child's impairment, where such exists, and the education environment are important factors in learning. In this way the two broad approaches can be married up. Norwich (1996) notes that the education field cannot avoid tensions between the two broad explanatory models and sets of values, but suggests that it is more useful in principle and practice to see the inter-relationships:

> 'the concept of SEN which has been connected with curriculum-based assessment cannot deny and avoid the importance of categories of impairment for meeting educational need' (Norwich, 1996: 102).

He suggests a compromise position whereby child differences can be recognised as interacting with education factors to influence educational need – his 'ideologically impure' approach, which incorporates both individual-personal and social-organisational perspectives. Such realistic approaches, which are also reflected in the code of practice (DfE, 1994) and the EPSEN document (SOEID, 1994), should help to overcome the functional barriers that can arise when teachers' and SLTs' models come into conflict, provided the underlying issues can be teased out and debated.

Models of collaboration across professions

The ways in which professionals construe their professional roles can help or hinder collaboration. So far this book has not attempted to define collaboration, but to take the discussion further some definition is needed.

Collaboration is clearly not an all-or-nothing phenomenon. Marvin (1990) presents a four-stage model, where only the highest level is labelled 'collaboration'.

Types of collaboration

co-activity, where professionals engage in separate teaching and learning
    activities, with little sharing of ideas. The analogy is made with children's
    parallel play
cooperation, where general goals are established jointly, but not goals for
    individual children
coordination, a form of group cohesion where the teacher and SLT share
    opinions and strategies relating to specific students, but do not actually
    work together
collaboration, where teachers and SLTs engage in informal networking, have
    a high degree of trust and respect for one another, and share responsi-
    bility for children

Marvin (1990)

DiMeo and colleagues (1998) also present a staged approach, and
suggest that cross-professional working is a developmental process, with
collaboration as the outcome of individuals learning to work together.
The need to foster good personal relationships is recognised in their
model, and although there can be movement from one level of working
together to another, not all SLT and teacher pairs are expected to achieve
collaborative partnerships. DiMeo and colleagues' model moves from a
stage they term *compliance* (where individuals interact on a minimal
level because they feel it is the professionally responsible thing to do), to
cooperation (where SLTs and teachers discuss and share ideas), to full
collaboration, where there is trust, respect and personal support
among professionals. They give examples of team teaching and joint
problem-solving approaches that result from good collaborative
practice.

These are very useful approaches, which recognise the variety of ways
in which SLTs and teachers work together to help children. The importance of social and interpersonal factors will be returned to. However,
for much of the discussion in this book a more general definition is
needed that allows consideration of less well-developed partnerships
under the broad heading of collaboration. The definition needs to be
sufficiently robust to encompass a variety of working settings and
practices but at the same time sufficiently clear to allow consideration of
whether a measure of collaborative working had been achieved or not.
Restricting the discussion to Marvin (1990) or DiMeo's (1998) highest
level would exclude much current practice.

The elements of sharing and working together appear to be the key
factors in most discussions of collaborative practice. For these reasons
the fairly 'strong' definition of collaboration offered by Conoley and
Conoley (1982) seems to meet the needs, and has already proved

productive in considerations of teachers' and SLTs' working practices (Kersner, 1996). Conoley and Conoley (1982) define collaboration as: 'the joining together of two or more individuals in an egalitarian relationship to achieve a mutually determined goal' (cited in Wright and Kersner, 1996: 34).

This definition of collaboration as requiring both joint goal planning and an equal relationship among colleagues seems to meet the requirements of an adequate working definition without restricting the discussion to thoroughly worked-out professional partnerships. The definition will therefore be used throughout the book to consider overall issues of interprofessional collaboration.

Either of the key factors contained in this working definition of collaboration can be omitted in current models of professional interaction: indeed, both can be. The 'transplant' model is discussed by McCool in Chapter 8 as being commonly used in health and education settings, where a professional owns the knowledge, skill and resources to help a child, while another individual acts as an 'aide' who has 'transplanted' only as much information as is needed to carry out some particular tasks. Goals are typically set by the professional. McCool discusses this issue in relation to work with parents, but teachers and therapists also employ this approach with others: teachers with classroom assistants, and SLTs with SLT assistants. Good relationships usually emerge, but neither of the factors needed for a collaborative partnership operates. A different working model is often used by a teacher or SLT acting as a student's placement supervisor, where joint planning between the student and professional may take place, but where the relationship is not egalitarian and the student benefits from the professional's greater experience. Certain medical teams, such as those involving a consultant and registrar, can operate in similar ways; such teams again may work well but do not meet both parameters of collaborative working.

A commonly used model of working in the health service is the construction of a multidisciplinary team (McGrath and Davis, 1992). In this model – which may involve for example paediatricians, physiotherapists, occupational therapists, SLTs and psychologists – professionals independently address a specific situation and create a forum where they meet and discuss their aims and objectives for the client. The partnerships are fairly egalitarian, although there is often a head of the team (often a physician!), but joint goals are not established. McGrath and Davis (1992) give further examples that they call interdisciplinary approaches, where objectives are set jointly by several disciplines, and Mackey and McQueen (1998) discuss an integrated therapy approach to family physiotherapy, which comes closer to the definition of collaboration used in this book.

Teachers and therapists may have different experiences of cross-disciplinary collaboration in different settings. McCaughey (1997a) reflected on her own recent move as an SLT from a child development centre in the health service to a language unit in a primary school. The child development centre could be characterised as operating a multidisciplinary model; the language unit as using a collaborative model between SLTs and teachers, but one where other professions were difficult to access and where parental contact with the unit was limited by location and transport problems. McCaughey reviews differences in practice resulting from the two models of intervention and discusses subtle differences in the types of joint planning that go on in the two settings.

Multidisciplinary and collaborative practice – contrasting examples

The needs of the child will dictate the type of intervention procedures offered by the therapist in a child development centre. This could be individual therapy, paired therapy sessions, group therapy or a combination of any of these models of service delivery. Treatment sessions may be provided jointly with other professionals from the team, and it is common practice for therapists from different disciplines to offer joint therapy sessions. The session's activities are jointly planned and a common shared activity is devised, to achieve each professional's therapy goal. However, although the therapy activity is shared, the professional goals are often different. Therefore this does not concur with Conoley and Conoley's (1982) definition of collaborative working, as the achievement of 'mutually determined goals', but it is an activity that has been collaboratively agreed upon and therefore it is not 'professionals independently addressing a specific situation' which de Lamerans-Pratt and Golden (1994) would define as multidisciplinary working. This suggests that there is a compromise common ground between multidisciplinary practices and collaborative approaches which is being utilised successfully by some professionals.

Intervention procedures in the language development unit are jointly planned and implemented. The programme of intervention is agreed and its implementation shared by the unit staff. At the end of each session, the staff of each classroom meet together to evaluate the day's work, to ensure that each member of the class team is kept informed of each individual child's daily progress (McCaughey, 1997: 5).

This suggests that in practice there are a wide variety of approaches to the issue of joint planning and, as Chapters 3 and 5 detail, various forms of joint planning are implemented. Fundamental assumptions about how professionals might interact will affect collaborative practice. The assumptions of SLTs and teachers in a working relationship about the underlying nature of that relationship may differ, or may simply be unexplored. Functional barriers to collaboration may occur where professionals are unwilling to discuss and clarify the professional interaction models operating, and to change them when they are not appropriate.

Social Barriers

Related to models of professional interaction is the fact that, because SLTs and teachers work for different organisations, when SLTs are in schools they are interacting with teacher colleagues who have little or no knowledge of the rest of their working context. There are some social difficulties inherent in being a 'visitor' in a school which apply to teachers such as learning support teachers as much as to SLTs and other professionals (Lovey, 1996). But in addition there are particular difficulties in belonging to a non-education profession, which were identified by Reid et al. (1996). Teachers unsurprisingly were not aware of SLTs' conditions of service, such as the fact that they had fewer weeks holiday than teachers and different working hours. SLTs tend not to be aware of how difficult it can be for teachers to leave a classroom, despite there being a number of sensible adults such as classroom assistants around, to discuss or observe SLTs' work. Although these seem trivial points, the consequences identified by Reid et al. (1996) were far from trivial, and misunderstandings affected good working relationships, perhaps inhibiting the 'mutual trust and respect' HMI (1996: 33) and DiMeo et al. (1998) identified as a hallmark of effective collaboration.

Structural Barriers

Structural barriers are related to the formalised ways in which each part of a service relates to other parts, dealing with relatively permanent and consistent aspects of the service. These can be considered as a priori, given features of the system which have to be considered by those operating in the service. In the context of the education and health systems, these include the timing and location of service delivery, management structures and curriculum structures. These will be discussed in turn.

Timing and location of service delivery

As well as fairly fundamental differences in service allocation, health and education differ in the times at which they make services accessible to clients. Schools have predetermined periods of the year and times of day at which classes will be taught, usually laid down by local authorities, and the timetable in the school day is often programmed ahead over long periods. Partly this is a matter of equality: since all children have to attend school, timing structures are a matter of organising holiday periods and starting times in an equitable way across a locality. They are not simply an administrative convenience, however: the amount of time a young child has to spend in school is a legal requirement, determined (from the start of compulsory education in the UK) to represent the optimum periods a child will spend in and out of school. Decisions are based on beliefs and knowledge about children's health and welfare.

The apparent rigidity in service timing derives from the fact that such decisions are made en masse for all children within an education authority's catchment area, and are backed up by legal requirements for their attendance.

SLT services are able to be more flexible, and endeavour to offer service at a time suitable to individual children's families. SLTs have agreed core guidelines and professional standards which comment on these issues, designed to help SLT services plan high-quality provision in a decentralised system. The guidelines state: 'All appointments should take into account ... the most mutually convenient location and time for the client' (RCSLT, 1996: 21).

SLT services are not restricted to school term times. However, as collaborative practices have come to the fore, SLTs have come to provide services in schools and therefore within school timetables. This has led to some difficulties if SLTs have their personal holidays during school terms, and teachers resent the loss of service at critical times in the school year. In expecting SLT services to accommodate to schools, schools are adopting some of the characteristics of a client, seeing that services are provided to the school rather than to the child. However, SLT services are more flexible and have endeavoured to accommodate such requests, for example by offering SLTs term-time contracts.

Location of service is also an issue. Schools are the location where education services are delivered to children. Schools are planned within a community in relation to the actual and predicted number of children in that locality, and education authorities provide transport for children if a school is situated outside a predetermined distance. Special education provision may involve further factors being taken into account in organising the number and location of schools, such as provision for specified disabilities across a larger geographical area, and will still make special transport arrangements. Education is therefore committed overall to providing a local service to be delivered in a convenient place.

SLT services also aim to provide a local and accessible service, and the professional guidelines state: 'An initial appointment will be offered at the nearest appropriate speech and language therapy location' (RCSLT, 1996: 21).

The low number of SLTs available has traditionally meant that SLTs have moved across wide geographical areas to provide staff in a number of locations. This can stretch SLT services. The example by Shaw and colleagues cited above at one time involved the SLT service in trying to provide cover to more than 70 schools, some of which had only one or two children requiring SLT input. The local health authority understandably questioned the efficiency of this expectation (Luscombe and Shaw, 1996: 9). Schools' commitments to local and inclusive services can put severe pressures on small SLT services, not due to any functional differences but due to structural factors. Grouping children differently can allow more intensive use of SLTs' time, and cut out wasted time, but this has to be set against the implications for the child's schooling. The problems probably result from resource limits more than any other factor, and as such are relatively intractable. These issues will be raised again in Chapter 6 where the particular difficulties of SLT collaboration in mainstream settings are discussed.

Despite these problems, SLT services have in recent years moved firmly into school settings. However, further location issues arise in the school itself. SLTs often prefer to work with children with language and communication difficulties on their own or in small groups, partly to avoid distraction for children who may have concentration and attention difficulties and partly because of the highly individual content of therapy programmes. It was no doubt an attempt to replicate the peace and privacy of these conditions that for many years prompted SLTs working in schools and units to withdraw children from classrooms and see them in private rooms in the school (HMI, 1996: 30, 31).

Collaborative work is, however, facilitated by working in classrooms, so that teachers and SLTs can actually work together. This does not allow much privacy, and although there are considerable compensating gains, SLTs may find working in the classroom difficult and distressing. Indeed, teachers may also find it difficult to accommodate another adult within the class, as evidence from learning support teachers suggests (Lovey, 1996).

A more fundamental difficulty for SLTs in the move to school-based work is the fact that the child in school is removed from the family setting, and opportunities to meet and work with parents may be limited compared with clinical settings. Reid et al. (1996: 77) reported that SLTs were concerned that a move from clinic-based to school-based services meant a lack of contact with parents, especially in mainstream school settings. Schools use a variety of meetings and written methods to keep in contact with parents, including parents evenings, but Reid's evidence was that SLTs were not routinely asked to these (Reid et al., 1996: 102). Once again, the change to collaborative work has costs as well as benefits, and these must be assessed carefully in order to be minimised.

Management Structures

Individual schools are part of a larger education system, where most of the other elements are schools, and where there is a recognised management hierarchy. In a school there is a headteacher responsible for the overall running of the school, often a deputy headteacher, and a number of classroom teachers, some with special responsibilities; including learning support teachers and, in England and Wales, special needs coordinators with a specific liaison role (Lacey, 1995). All of these people, and most of the people in the wider education sector, will share the profession of teacher, and will have undergone similar training programmes to enter that profession. Even on their pre-service qualifying courses and degree programmes teachers may have had limited opportunity to interact with other professionals in training, and SLT students may similarly have had few experiences of learning alongside student teachers.

Schools are set in an education authority context where national and local policies are developed to facilitate their organisation and running. Such policy is subject to public influence via local authority representation, but is developed largely in association with schools and education officers who have themselves trained as teachers. Similarly, learning support teachers are appropriately drawn from the teaching profession. Teachers on the whole meet and work with teachers, where they can reasonably assume some shared attitudes and experiences, but may have limited experience of working in cross-professional groups.

SLTs on the other hand work in NHS trusts where the number of SLTs employed may be small and where the therapy services director may be from another profession (Mays and Pope, 1997). This would be a very unusual circumstance in education: Miller (1994) draws an analogy with a school from which the headteacher had been removed and a senior chiropodist appointed as manager. SLTs conform to local and national policies pertaining to the health service, but these are designed to influence many professions and are not specifically targeted to SLTs.

This management structure, together with relative autonomy in planning the timing and location of service delivery as discussed above, means that an individual SLT has usually acted as an independent professional, responsible for selecting which clients will be seen, and when, and where, and for how long. Such individual negotiation of how a client load will be managed has in turn provided families (as surrogate clients for their young children) with a sense of control over the amount, type and timing of SLT intervention. The small number of SLTs has limited flexibility to those times and places where an SLT was available, but the appearance of individual control is strong.

In these ways, individual SLTs operate rather like a whole school. SLTs are used to working with a variety of professions and parents in ways which teachers may not be, but are unused to sharing decisions about individual children and therapy plans. Working together will be affected by these structures – teachers being asked to share classrooms with other professions perhaps for the first time; SLTs losing independence of action on some decisions. Such differences, badly handled, will again provide barriers to collaboration.

Curriculum Structures

After extensive debate and discussion, the countries which comprise the UK have nationwide curricula in place covering the school years to adolescence: the National Curriculum in England, Wales and Northern Ireland and the 5–14 Curriculum in Scotland. Details of curricular approaches will no doubt alter and be adapted over time, refined by the distillation of good practice across the country, but the idea that there will continue to be nationally agreed curricula appears to be settled. Debate has moved on to the best mechanisms for delivery of the curriculum, and how to ensure excellence of standards in the school system. Consideration is given to how individual children may access this curriculum, and how to address any special learning needs they may have, but the right of every child to access the curriculum is enshrined in law and in school practices (DfEE, 1997). This is now the systems environment in which schools operate, and the curriculum itself has become a structural aspect of school organisation.

SLTs have had no such central direction about what language and communication skills to develop, or how to approach intervention. They once again make individual decisions, and many of the questions about how best to influence children's language disorders have yet to receive satisfactory answers, although there is evidence of the overall effectiveness of a variety of intervention approaches (Law et al., 1998). SLT services therefore rely on published examples of good practice, and on research studies into intervention programmes and plans. These are sometimes used on an agreed basis by SLTs throughout a whole SLT service, but there are no practices that are comparable to the UK national curricula.

Such differences between school and SLT perceptions of the centrality of a curriculum can create tensions for SLTs and teachers who want to work in partnership. Teachers will probably want to plan language in the curriculum and may see the end point of language teaching as improved access to the school curriculum. This may seem a restrictive aim to SLTs, who are used to constructing aims and goals in terms of improved communication in all aspects of a child's life, including home and social contexts. The school in their model is only one example of a social context, albeit an important one. If the aim of language education is to help a child's attainment of curriculum goals and targets, this can seem to ignore much of a child's real-life experience. The emphasis in the school curriculum on talking and listening has been an important mechanism for fostering collaboration, but many SLTs may not immediately see the relevance of planning in a curriculum framework.

There are also difficulties in matching curricular and SLT models of language. SLTs typically use developmental approaches, assessing children's progress along the continuum followed by all children in acquiring language, and matching language goals to the next stage of developmental progression. Daines (1992) points out that the ways in which the (English and Welsh) national curriculum approaches language are very different, being developmentally insensitive and at times using examples of target language attainments that are used by much younger children in the home context.

Furthermore, as Daines also comments, the national curriculum looks at language largely in terms of the functions and use of language. SLTs are often concerned with helping children improve language forms such as speech sound systems and grammar. This is particularly because many children have intelligibility problems and because difficulty with aspects of language form (especially the verb phrase) distinguishes children with specific language disorders from their peers (Rice and Wexler, 1996). Since the national curricula are concerned largely with educating normally developing children who will have mastered most language forms before they reach school, their emphasis on language use is entirely appropriate. However, for many children with language and communication difficulties, curricular aims concerned with language use may not seem to meet their needs. The Association for all Speech Impaired Children (AFASIC), a voluntary society concerned with the needs of children with language and communication difficulties, makes this point, commenting that children with language difficulties need specialised help and often: 'must be taught the skills of using speech and language which the unimpaired acquire without such help' (AFASIC, 1990: 1).

Agreeing joint goals may be further impeded by the fact that it is in the area of language form that teachers and SLTs have a mismatch of knowledge. SLTs have highly developed assessment and intervention techniques to target language forms based on linguistic analysis, but Miller (1991) found that teachers, who have usually considered the needs of children over the age of 5 years, require much more information on normal language development and assessment to help them work with children who have difficulties.

Although SLTs as 'outsiders' in the school context may be most forcibly struck by such tensions between the overt assumptions of the curriculum and the child's perceived needs, teachers have also signalled reservations about too much reliance on the curriculum. Respondents to the National Council for the Curriculum's review of special education needs (NCC, 1993) made similar points:

Teachers point out that, for all pupils with special education needs ... the National Curriculum provides only part of the curriculum. Access to developmental work across the curriculum, personal and social education and enrichment activities in particular, should be given equal status with access to National Curriculum subjects and religious education. It is a question of getting the balance or the context right (p. 2).

If curricular stages and assessments become too much of a strait-jacket, planning joint goals in the school curriculum can become another barrier to collaboration. However, the examples in the next chapter suggest that good collaboration has in practice been achieved where SLTs and teachers have accepted the need to adapt strong curricular structures to reflect the needs of the child, and to adopt the curriculum as the basis but not the end point of joint planning.

Process Barriers

A process model focuses on how a system behaves, and in this context considers the ways in which SLT and school services organise contact with children and their families. Focusing on the child, and taking a simple event sequence, process models allow discussion of the ways in which a child can access services, how progress is reviewed and how transfer to other services is organised. This model is useful in considering how services serve children. The principal means of organising these processes in education services is by considering a statement or record of special education needs, and this will be discussed. The main issues revolve around whether or not a full statement or record is opened, and the involvement of school and SLT services in maintaining and reviewing the process.

Opening a statement or record of special educational needs

The context in which SLTs and education services collaborate in setting up a statement or record of special educational needs is outlined in Chapter 1, and differences in funding SLT input are mentioned. The decision about when it is appropriate to set up a statement or record will be further clarified and amended by policy debate at governmental and local level.

The complexity and expense of opening a statement or record of special educational needs can be seen as a barrier to accessing services, in that the effort needed to open and maintain the statement or record can in itself divert resources from meeting educational needs. Such factors mean that most children's needs should properly be dealt with in schools without a full record or statement being opened. However, there is a great deal of local variation in whether a child receives statement or record (DfEE, 1997). In relation to children with language and communication difficulty, the Scottish HMI (1996), having reviewed specialist provision for children with language and communication difficulties across Scotland, commented on this unexplained variation, noting:

> The majority of pupils attending separate special schools had Records of Needs. Of the remaining pupils in pre-school or primary units, 30% had

Records of Needs. In one unit all the pupils were recorded but in the other units the proportion of those who were recorded varied substantially (p. 14).

Since there appeared to be no satisfactory explanation for such variation, HMI went on to make a strong statement about the need to record all children whose speech, language or communication disorders result in pronounced, specific or complex special needs which were persistent and likely to require continuing review (HMI, 1996: 14, 35). Such children are likely to require SLT input. Policy in England and Wales seems to be accepting the need for some national criteria while reducing the overall number of children with statements (DfEE, 1997). Clarification and guidelines would be useful, but the overall thrust of education policy suggests that most children with language and communication disorders will not receive a statement or record.

As Chapter 1 discusses, there is a particular issue concerning collaboration and the opening of a statement or record of special needs because of different funding for SLT input. In Scotland, where differential funding is most highly developed, the situation whereby it can seem easier for a child with a record of special educational needs to access SLT services has led to a 'rush to record' (Reid et al., 1996: 78), and to open a record specifying SLT and other services. This is related to resources and educational factors. Whereas educationists worry that the process of opening a statement or record will 'clog up' the system, and perhaps stigmatise children unnecessarily, Reid et al. (1996: 74) found that SLT managers worried that as more children are recorded annually but not discharged, and as inflation eroded the value of education funding for SLT services, it would not be possible to maintain levels of SLT input to education. Issues around the opening of a statement or record of special education needs can cause collaboration problems if the demand for services once again outstrips supply, and where pressures to secure SLT input conflict with pressures to open records or statements only when it is essential to do so. SLT services are concerned to maintain satisfactory levels of service to the majority of children who will not receive a record or statement, and can resent their input to clients being controlled so closely by education interests.

Planning for special education needs

In a process model, consideration can be given to the ways in which services are offered to individual children. Schools and SLT services both advocate processes involving a review of a child's needs and the formation of a plan to structure learning experiences to meet these needs, followed by further reviews. Here, there appears to be a clear concordance between the professions, and few barriers to collaboration.

Subsequent chapters will describe how SLT and school services work together to deliver high-quality services to children, despite barriers. The key to this may be the fundamental agreement between the two professions on the processes to be adopted to help children learn, rather than the legal procedures involved in noting such agreement.

There is an expectation in education that children engaged in a differentiated curriculum will have an IEP that details individually relevant adaptations to the curriculum. Despite some functional difficulties, there is no particular tension between SLT services and school services in such approaches – both professions are usually happy to spell out their aims and objectives for a particular child, and how they will set about achieving them. SLTs are familiar with measuring the outcomes of intervention, often measured as language gains and sometimes including comparison with normally developing children. Teachers are also familiar with measuring curriculum attainments, and with tracking children's progress through education tasks such as reading and maths schemes. Both professions can often see the benefits of sharing and eventually amalgamating their plans, and indeed in a collaborative approach an IEP can incorporate the aims of all professions and give details of how these are to be implemented.

In considering process measures, therefore, there seem to be fewer tensions between SLTs and teachers than are seen at other levels in the health and education systems, once the difficult decisions around the opening of a statement or record of needs are taken. This is a hopeful conclusion, and paves the way for the argument that much good collaborative practice can flourish 'on the ground'.

Systems-environment barriers

The systems-environment model is used to consider school and SLT services in the context of the community and of the larger society: Banathy's (1992) 'bird's-eye view of the landscape' in which the system is sited. Such an outlook encourages questions about how adequately a service responds to the context in which it is set and, conversely, about how responsive that context is to the service that is on offer. In the case of schools and SLT services the field could be very wide, and some influences of overall education and health service systems have already been considered. It would be possible to look beyond these to social and cultural factors operating on services, and the mediating effect of government and local policies. There is, however, the more immediate issue of children's families to be considered, and the relationships with parents assumed by each service and developed in service provision. The systems-environment model could also be developed to take account of children's perspectives, but for the purposes of this book families will be considered to be surrogate service users.

Families and Services

Parents, carers and families are formally welcomed as partners in both education and health services, as reflected in statutory and professional policies (HMI, 1996; RCSLT, 1996; DfEE, 1997). They are recognised as playing a key role when considering a child's language needs, and are involved in all formal decisions about school placement and opening and maintaining statements or records of need. Their role in further forms of decision-making may vary from service to service, but the importance of fostering a positive and mutually supportive relationship between service, child and carer is universally agreed. McCool in Chapter 8 discusses the roles parents are encouraged to adopt in school and therapy services, and the implications for service delivery and development.

The ways in which schools and SLT services organise interactions with families are rather different. Schools are set up in part to help children as they grow and develop to function without constant parental support, and at times schools must counteract the effects of maladaptive family practices. However, school services want to involve parents in education processes, and to foster purposeful relationships. To do this, as discussed earlier, they have to timetable contact with families in a fairly formal manner, and may not be able to accommodate family preferences. Some specialist provisions such as language units may not be particularly local, and the fact that children are escorted to school by special transport may further mean that face-to-face contact between parents and school staff is difficult to organise (although telephone contacts, taxi escorts and home–school diaries can serve a useful liaison function). The relative formality of patterns of contact may be off-putting to parents. They are usually included in formal, annual review meetings in school to discuss their child's progress, ideally supported by written reports in advance, but HMI (1996: 31) noted that some parents were intimidated by such large cross-disciplinary conferences. Some parents have input to planning their children's programmes in schools but this is not universal: Reid et al. (1996: 102) noted that less than half of the parents of children with language and communication difficulties they interviewed were involved in deciding on children's therapy plans, but less than one-fifth had been included in devising an IEP or in decisions about education programmes.

Therapy services have traditionally had rather different patterns of contact with parents, and because of the developmental nature of language and communication difficulties, families may have had extensive contact with SLT services before the child enters school or nursery. Many such services will be based in local community settings that will have welcomed parents into therapy sessions to discuss plans and activities for their child in detail. Many parents will have carried out tasks in the home setting designed to help their children's language development, and some will have attended groups and workshops designed to support parents in developing useful interaction strategies. Many will have had experience of multidisciplinary teams operating in child development centres or specialist hospital settings, where the family is the focus of intervention approaches. Because of this early involvement, parents may well have met a health service and SLT model of individual or small group working before they meet school practices. They may also have met 'medical' models of children's disabilities, and services selected and targeted at those who could best benefit, and will have seen their children receive services in this context.

Furthermore, if parents have internalised the individualised, health service model as an ideal model of how an SLT service should operate, it may be difficult to convince them of the benefits of a different model of service delivery as practised in schools. Even when good collaboration occurs between teachers and SLTs, parents may feel excluded and confused about the service being offered to their child. McCaughey (1997b) discussed such issues in detail with one set of parents. They had considerable experience of services delivered to themselves and their child via a child development centre, and their son had recently moved to a part-time pre-school nursery placement in a language development unit. The parents gave a balanced account of both types of service for their developing child (further outlined in Chapter 3), and were pleased overall with the provision he was receiving. None the less, the mother commented that, although she knew that for three of the four days a week her child spent in the nursery the SLT was in his class, she was unsure of the amount of therapy he received, and was concerned that it might be less than in the child development centre.

The question of what constitutes 'real' SLT services for parents may prove a barrier to collaboration. If parents' models of therapy remain the one-to-one SLT-to-child model, collaborative models may be seen as less focused and less intensive by parents. Services wishing to adopt a collaborative approach will have to explain their context and rationale for service provision with care, and to be prepared that parents might resist such explanations. The environment in which SLT and school services operate may be more sympathetic to health service ways of working with children than to schools', at least as far as children's families are concerned. If parents' experiences have led them to internalise a 'medical' model of understanding their children's difficulties, perhaps using a diagnostic label and clinical classification, they can feel that their perspectives are being ignored when schools concentrate on curriculum learning needs. This is somewhat ironic, as this education approach is designed to lead to helpful actions which many educationists feel are not facilitated by medical classifications. The dual approach of Norwich (1996), referred to above, might be helpful to use in discussion with parents.

Conclusion

The differences in systems outlined above can give rise to difficulties in practice. This chapter has spelled out the differences, on the assumption that listing the inherent tensions places them on an agenda for debate and change. However, many of the structural, functional and systems-environment barriers that exist between health service and education systems seem set to remain for some time. The two systems will proceed in parallel, and those working in them may at times be confused by the assumptions and practices of the other service. The value of addressing differences may therefore be to allow SLTs and teachers reciprocal access to the other profession's fundamental models, to allow mutual understanding and sharing of the opportunities and constraints that result.

The systems approach used suggests that there are fewer barriers in operation at the level of process than at other systems levels, and that the systems in place at the level of planning for the school child can minimise potential problems if used effectively. Dessent (1996: 16) makes a similar observation, noting that at his 'casework/fieldwork' level involving collaborative assessment and provision for individual children and families:

> teacher, speech therapist [sic], nursery nurse, doctor and psychologist work co-operatively and in partnership with parents to plan, deliver and monitor intervention programmes. Successful working of this kind occurs in thousands of situations daily. ... All of these activities take place each day blissfully unaffected by the obstacles previously listed.

This chapter has argued that collaborative practice is not unaffected by systems obstacles, and that these remain serious barriers. However, there are equally serious attempts to overcome these taking place. Child-based processes already provide an essential point of contact for the services, and this perhaps explains why so much good collaborative practice is being developed, as detailed in the next few chapters. As these examples will show, collaboration has occurred mainly through SLTs accepting the school system as the operating context, and adapting their procedures and practices to fit in with school expectations. In this they are operating as purpose-seeking systems, seeking an ideal of service delivery and evolving with the current environment (Banathy, 1996: 272–3). However, such services run the risk that they will not be well understood by their health service colleagues and managers. A great deal of explanation and mutual sharing will continue to be required if good collaborative practice is to further develop.

Chapter 3
Patterns of Collaboration

ELSPETH McCARTNEY

Introduction

Chapter 2 discussed difficulties and barriers to collaboration between SLTs and teachers, but found considerable common ground at the process level of planning for an individual child. Some barriers existed even at that level, and there were considerable obstacles reflected in all systems models. However, the aims of both schools and SLT services are to help children to talk and listen effectively, and there is recognition that good professional collaboration can facilitate this process. SLTs and teachers have therefore been developing ways of collaboration that try to overcome the barriers identified in Chapter 2. Evidence of good collaboration comes from the literature, from research and from practical examples of recent practice. This chapter will summarise such evidence, using the headings and systems approaches developed in earlier chapters to suggest how barriers to collaboration are being overcome, and to illustrate good practice.

Patterns of collaboration fit into Banathy's systems approaches as outlined in earlier chapters. The development of policy statements will be considered using the functions model, which considers the goals and purposes of collaboration and collaborative practice. The formalised ways in which services are organised to work with children with language difficulties will be examined using the structures model, and processes will be examined to consider the dynamic interaction between the SLT and education systems. Systems-environment influences are extensive, and could include context-setting factors such as parents' organisations, research and those concerned with the maintenance of standards such as Ofsted and HMI. However, the environmental influence that most affects collaboration is probably the child's immediate family, and so the focus will be on work with parents. For all four systems, the issues discussed in Chapter 2 will be revisited in order to consider how barriers to collaboration are being overcome, and to give some illustrative examples. Later chapters of the book take up these issues in more detail, presenting further reviews and examples of good practice.

Functional Issues

In Chapter 1 barriers were identified concerning the goals and purposes of services, including which children should be prioritised, the interaction of children's disabilities with curriculum adaptations, and issues of interprofessional collaboration. Solutions and partial solutions to such barriers can be identified, and have been incorporated in policy statements and good practice models in a variety of settings.

Collaboration in selecting and prioritising children

Two related problems were identified in Chapter 2 concerning selecting and prioritising children. One was the fundamental difference between education as an allocating service, providing services to all children of school age, as opposed to health, which is a commissioning and rationing service, dealing only with individuals who have an identified need. This means that SLT services do not have the responsibility of developing the language and communication skills of all children, which remains a principal goal of education services. This distinction between the functions of services remains, and may cause particular difficulties for SLTs and early educationalists working in pre-school and reception classes. Because children develop language skills at different rates, there are problems in predicting which children will have persisting difficulties (Bishop and Edmundson, 1987). Many children with early difficulties, particularly those with no verbal comprehension problems, catch up fairly well with their peers during childhood (Paul et al., 1997). There can be difficulties for SLT services in justifying work with young children, and in balancing the expected benefits of early intervention with the need to use resources effectively (Law, 1997). Educationalists, on the other hand, argue firmly for offering the benefits of early education to all, which has led to a recent expansion of nursery provision and a focus on the early school years.

As children move through the school years, however, any speech, language and communication difficulties will usually be overt, particularly if they are in the area of language form, where most developmental processes should be complete. Decisions about access to special services are then handled by both education and SLT services in similar ways, by establishing the child's individual and distinctive needs and planning actions to meet these. In this way, both services become prioritising services, and the second problem can arise if SLTs and teachers fail to agree on priorities and actions.

It is often appropriate that SLT and education services make separate decisions about which children should receive special help from each service. For example, a child with specific speech difficulties may be making good progress in the school curriculum, while requiring SLT input to help with intelligibility. Discussions between the SLT and teacher about what to do if the child is not understood in class and about the demands made by a reading scheme will be useful, but the child could appropriately be prioritised by the SLT service and not the school. Similarly, children with educational and behavioural difficulties may have no language or communication problems that require attention by the SLT, but require a whole-school approach to help them to learn. There are many such instances where separate decision making is appropriate, but language and communication difficulties are so pervasive and have such an adverse effect on learning that joint decision making may more commonly be required.

The recognition by NHS trusts and education authorities of the need for joint decisions on service provision has led to forward planning to try to determine the number of children who might require services, and to plan the funding of SLT services in schools, as recommended by HMI (1996: 42). This will involve SLT services and education authorities taking account of the special education needs of pupils, the views of parents and professionals, and local circumstances. HMI suggests that the provision of educational psychologists and occupational therapists should also be reviewed. Reid et al. (1996: 107) make similar suggestions about an evaluation of need, suggesting specifically that educational psychology services could estimate the annual number of children in their area who have SLT provision listed as a requirement in their record of needs. This would provide a 'formula' for predicting the provision of SLT services at a local level. SLT managers should also make an input into discussions among associations of education authorities and at regional and national health service planning levels to consider budgetary aspects of provision (Reid et al., 1996: 74).

In Scotland, as Chapter 1 outlined, such a formula could be used by education authorities to purchase SLT services directly. In the rest of the UK it would help predict what resources local trusts would need to find for SLT funding, and would help create a national picture which would feed into requirements for staffing and service provision.

Consideration of the functions of collaboration has therefore led to the need to predict the amount of collaborative work to be undertaken, its costs and funding. This should feed into considerations of structure and local, national and regional systems for predicting and contracting for SLT services.

Collaboration in models of practice

Chapter 2 outlined another fundamental difference between education and health services, where education services were concerned mainly with curriculum adaptations and SLTs were partly concerned with identifying and attempting to 'fix' a child's difficulties. It also referred to Norwich's (1996) arguments which develop a third approach, one that recognises the duality of the issue. He considers that settling on any single explanatory model and set of values can unhelpfully restrict diversity of perspectives, and recognises that both approaches offer valid considerations. A dual approach allows, among other things, some prediction of the likely long-term or short-term nature of a child's special needs, and clarifies the purposes of assessment in the identification of learning difficulties and special educational needs. MacKay and Anderson make similar points in Chapter 4, and a dual perspective is also implicit in the English and Welsh Code of Practice (DfE, 1994) and the Scottish EPSEN report (SOEID, 1994); both of which emphasise the need for gathering information on any impairments such as language and communication difficulties when planning adapted provision.

Such a dual approach to the functions of collaborative work can provide an impetus for teachers and SLTs to interact purposefully. There is clearly a role for teachers in understanding the curriculum and knowing the variety of ways in which learning objectives can be facilitated. There is a role for SLTs in assessing within frameworks of language and communication disability to help clarify where a child's difficulties lie. However, these roles can, and probably should, also be reversed, so that teachers assess children's communication in the classroom and with peers, and SLTs observe learning characteristics and consider ways in which materials can be presented. Mackay and Young in Chapter 5 and MacKinnon (1997) below outline joint assessment procedures that parallel independent professional assessments to form the basis for useful collaborative planning. Popple and Wellington (1996) give examples working in a psycholinguistic framework.

However, the historical tendency for educationalists to concentrate on curriculum matters and for SLTs to consider child difficulties may mean that SLTs and teachers in practice have limited knowledge in the reciprocal area. Miller (1991) surveyed teachers in the UK teaching children with speech and language difficulties and asked what further information they felt they needed. Among their priorities were to have 'a language to talk about language' and to know how to talk about speech and language difficulties with parents and professionals. Roux (1996) asked newly qualified SLTs what they wanted to know about working in schools. Many of their problems centred around role definition (worries about being expected to demonstrate 'expert' status which they did not profess), but they also needed to increase their own knowledge and understanding of the curriculum and teaching methods.

The solution to this need to share information is often found in joint training and inservice sessions that attempt to 'fill the gaps' and explain one profession's frameworks to the other. Jeans et al. (1997) surveyed mainstream school teachers in their locality about the information they required. About three-quarters of the 64 respondents wanted further information on local SLT services (such as range of services, referral criteria, criteria for mainstream support, information about the local clinic and procedures following referral) and most wanted inservice training for their staff. The range of inservice topics (presented below in rank order) confirmed Miller's (1991) earlier work, being concerned with aspects of language and language development which are not covered in the curriculum but which are relevant to the difficulties shown by language-disordered children.

Mainstream teachers' inservice requirements
By rank order:
- speech sound development
- linguistic concept development
- play and language development
- auditory memory difficulties
- language disorders including the autistic continuum
- attention control
- stammering.

Jeans et al. (1997: 12)

Roux's (1996) examples (not rank-ordered) of the needs for support of new therapists in schools give a parallel list:

SLTs' inservice requirements
- revisiting theoretical issues using the SLT's experience
- reflecting on positive experiences and identifying factors that facilitated them
- support for working with parents in school
- information on assessment methods and opportunities in the school setting
- information on working within the curriculum (including a knowledge of the curriculum and teaching methods)
- information on the development of literacy and numeracy skills
- the management of collaboration
  - joint planning
  - joint goal setting
  - joint intervention
- suggestions about how to increase opportunities for liaison (including time management)
- consideration of working with other professionals in school
  - learning support assistants
  - classroom assistants
  - educational psychologists
  - bilingual co-workers
- understanding the issues involved in inclusive education and equal access and entitlement with reference to SLT services.

Roux (1996: 56-7)

Such lists can provide useful frameworks for devising surveys of training needs and planning joint courses. Continuing professional development is clearly needed, and joining SLTs and teachers in shared inservice programmes can be an efficient and effective way of kick-starting and developing collaborative working.

Models of interprofessional collaboration

In Chapter 2 a distinction was made between 'strong' collaborative approaches, with joint planning in equal partnerships, and multidisciplinary approaches, where teachers and SLTs planned separately and had different goals, but shared information about progress. The 'transplant' model was also outlined, where one member of the team 'owned' the knowledge and required skill to tackle a problem, and transferred only as much as necessary to another team member to allow specific tasks to be carried out (McCool in Chapter 8 gives further details). Marvin's (1990) and DiMeo et al.'s (1998) staged approaches were outlined, and subtle combinations of these approaches in practice were discussed by McCaughey (1997a). As collaborative approaches develop we would expect to see a range of ways in which SLTs and teachers work together.

Different models have been adopted to suit differing circumstances, and the ways in which professionals collaborate have gradually been refined over time. It is possible to seek evidence for 'strong' collaboration models in recent policy statements, both in education and in the SLT profession, which set frameworks and strongly influence practice. The origins of such statements in separate public service systems tends to result in either health or education being taken as the defining context, and, by their nature, policy statements give few examples of just how skills and expertise are to be shared. The overall recognition of the need for SLTs and teachers to work together is, however, clearly expressed.

Education policies on collaboration

Government departments of education both in England and Wales and in Scotland have produced policy documents that refer to collaboration between teachers and SLTs.

In England and Wales, the code of practice on the identification and assessment of special education needs (DfE, 1994) outlines the need for LEAs to ensure that SLTs' advice has been sought in planning to meet the SENs of children, including children with speech and language difficulties. The cognate EPSEN document in Scotland (SOEID, 1994) makes similar arrangements. Education policy guidance documents also refer to collaborative working when presenting materials designed to help planning for SENs within the curriculum. A good example comes from

SOED (1993), where the key roles of staff, including 'support services from outwith the school' are discussed, with SLTs included as offering support to the teacher rather than services to the child. This implies a measure of collaboration, which is made more explicit when specifying the roles to be played by SLTs. The document states:

> Class and learning support teachers are assisted in planning language work for pupils with language and communications difficulties by receiving guidance and advice from these therapists. In specialist provision speech and language therapists collaborate with teachers in planning, implementing and evaluating programmes of study (Part I: 25).

This makes a distinction between 'strong' collaboration in specialist provision, where joint planning can be expected to take place, and a weaker model in mainstream settings where SLTs are given rather more of the 'expert' role of providing guidance and advice to classroom and support teachers. This distinction will be discussed further in Chapter 6. No examples of how collaboration is to be achieved are given, but the same document suggests that school policies will wish to detail the services provided from outside the school (such as SLT) and the arrangements for integrating these contributions within classrooms and in IEPs (Part II: 22).

Further guidance to schools in working with SLTs as 'specialist support services' appears in the Scottish EPSEN document (SOEID, 1994), which considers effective provision, and the more limited English and Welsh Code of Practice (DfE, 1994), which is concerned largely with identification and assessment of need. The EPSEN document gives further guidance on the role of the headteacher and class teacher in working with other professionals including SLTs. Headteachers are to agree with each professional arrangements to facilitate his or her work and that of the school, and to ensure that class teachers understand the roles of the specialists and the expectations of working together. They are also to make consultation time between class teachers and specialists available, with parents present where appropriate, and arrange for class teachers to be trained by specialists where appropriate. Class teachers are to agree priorities for pupils and integrate specialist activities into the child's work programme (SOEID, 1994: 46). This document still hints at a model in which SLTs extract children from the classroom: class teachers are urged to adjust timetables to ensure that specialists are able to work with pupils when they are not distracted or missing important lessons (p. 47). The overall emphasis however reflects a positive approach, promoting the idea of a coordinated multidisciplinary team and emphasising communication, commitment and evaluation.

These ideas are further developed in more recent policy. In a report that looks specifically and extensively at services to children with language and communication disorders in Scotland, HMI (1996) stress 'sound partnership' between speech and language therapists and teachers (p. 39) as a necessary requirement of effective provision for such pupils, and devotes a section to describing how such partnerships can be fostered. There is an emphasis on cognitive and emotional aspects of professionals working together, as stressed also by DiMeo et al. (1998), as well as the sharing of knowledge and information.

Hallmarks of good collaboration
HMI list the 'hallmarks' of good collaboration as:

- mutual trust and respect, where teachers and SLTs have confidence in each other and respect each other's expertise
- joint goal setting, where language goals are drawn up together by teachers and SLTs, consulting as necessary
- joint training, so that the perspectives, knowledge base and priorities of the other profession can be explored
- parental satisfaction with the provision.

(HMI, 1996: 39)

This is a statement advocating strong collaboration, emphasising the com-plementary roles of the professionals involved, and stressing joint planning and execution of plans. It implies a move away from the SLT as 'specialist' or 'support service' and recognises the centrality of both the teacher and the SLT in helping children. The green paper (DfEE, 1997) makes similar points. Such a step-change in education policy is to be welcomed.

SLT policies on collaboration

The SLT profession also makes commitments to collaboration in its professional standards document (RCSLT, 1996). This document differentiates between mainstream and specialist schools, but the need for strong collaboration is stressed in both settings.

SLT aims in mainstream schools are:

1   To provide a service that involves a high degree of shared knowledge, skills, expertise and information among all those involved with the child.
2   To provide speech and language therapy assessment and intervention for children with speech and language difficulties as an integral part of their school life, ensuring that speech and language therapy input is part of a total programme for the child.
3   To recognise and implement highly flexible working practices with the focus on the everyday social and learning context of the child
4   To acknowledge that a speech and language therapy service in a mainstream school is a specialist service and not simply a speech and language therapy 'clinic' located in a school.

> 5   To deliver the service in such a way as to enable education staff to incor-
> porate the aims of the speech and language therapy programme in the
> context of the broad curriculum.
>
> RCSLT (1996: 54)

All these aims imply collaborative practice, although the fifth aim suggests some independent planning, with the curriculum as the vehicle for accessing the 'speech and language therapy programme', rather than vice versa.

In discussing provision in special schools and language units, similar points are made, but with a greater emphasis on collaboration.

> **SLT aims in special schools are:**
>
> 1   To provide assessment and intervention for children with communica-
> tion and/or eating and drinking difficulties as part of their education life.
> 2   To deliver the service in such a way as to enable the education staff to
> incorporate the aims of the speech and language therapy programme
> into the language curriculum for each child with a speech and language
> difficulty.
> 3   To work with the school staff, carers and other professionals to facilitate
> the child's development, to carry out specific therapy where appro-
> priate, to serve as a resource for the school staff in preparing any school
> policies and to be available as a resource for relevant areas of the
> curriculum.
> 4   To contribute to workshops for staff and carers on topics relating to
> communication and/or eating and drinking.
>
> RCSLT (1996: 57)

For language units, aims are even more overtly concerned with collaborative approaches, and have recognised that 'ownership' of the programme to help the child involves education issues.

> **SLT aims in language units are:**
>
> 1   To provide a service that involves a high degree of shared knowledge,
> skills, expertise and information among those involved with the child.
> 2   To provide speech and language support, assessment and intervention
> for the child attending the unit as an integral part of school life. This
> would ensure that speech and language therapy input is implicit in the
> child's education programme, acknowledging that ownership of the
> programme is with the education authority.
> 3   To recognise that primacy of care is with the education authority for the
> holistic management of the child's speech and language difficulties.
> 4   To implement working practices that accommodate all the needs of the
> child, in addition to those needs specifically identified by the speech and
> language therapist's assessment.

5   To acknowledge that education placement in a language unit recognises that the child's speech and language difficulties have implications for his/her education, and that a positive statement is being made about the child's overall needs being intrinsic to his/her speech and language needs.

6   To deliver the service in such a way as to work with the education staff, incorporating the aims of the speech and language therapy programme in the planning of the language programme.

RCSLT (1996: 61)

These are very positive statements about collaborative practice, although they do recognise some separate 'therapy programme' which could at least be differentiated from the overall plan for a child. The SLT professional standards document (RCSLT, 1996) goes on to detail how an interface and liaison with other professionals are to be achieved. In relation to mainstream settings, the need for SLTs to acknowledge their role as members of a multidisciplinary team and to recognise the primacy of the child's education needs is detailed. The need to share expertise and to develop confidence in education staff who work with the child is stressed, as is the need to establish multidisciplinary links. This goes beyond the role of expert and advice giver, for example by assuming some responsibility for sharing knowledge and skills with teachers, but does not explicitly identify joint planning as an essential component of the service.

When working in special schools and language units, the professional guidelines repeat these points, but add to the list the need to share skills and roles in a collaborative way. The need for formalised discussion time is stressed, as is the need to meet parents and others concerned with the child to ensure a holistic approach to overall planning. There is thus a formal commitment from the SLT profession to work in a collaborative manner, and some examples are given of how this is to be accomplished.

Linking policy on interprofessional collaboration

The thrust of the policy statements from both education and SLT systems is to stress the need for joint working. In settings where the education needs of the child are focused around language difficulty, such as language units and special schools, the statements on collaboration are stronger and better developed. Where children are in mainstream schools, the need for collaboration is also recognised, but models are less strong. This point will be returned to in Chapter 6, and perhaps reflects the more limited opportunities for collaboration in mainstream settings, where there may be only a few children receiving SLT input in any one school.

The model of a strongly collaborative service is held in policy statements as the ideal model, and one that is being attained in a number of settings. Policy on good working practice has become clear, and is in sympathy with many practitioners' aims and opinions. The barriers that exist are being seen as practical constraints to be overcome rather than as boundaries to be preserved. Given the historical variety of models of professional interaction that have existed both within and between SLT and school services, this is a considerable achievement.

Social interaction

The lack of understanding of the whole working context of the teacher by the SLT, and vice versa, can prove a barrier to collaboration (Roux, 1996). Such a lack of understanding can militate against the mutual trust and respect noted by HMI as a hallmark of good collaborative practice, and at a practical level can prevent teachers and SLTs from knowing who to contact and how to access one another. Some of the structural ways of organising services, such as specialist teams of SLTs going into particular schools, may be useful in forging better social links, as would joint inservice training as discussed above and advocated by HMI (1996) and earlier by David and Smith (1991). Just being together in the same work context may, however, be the best mechanism for developing shared understanding and rewarding social interactions. Mainstream school settings may once again prove to be difficult settings in view of the limited time spent there by any SLT, with special schools and language units being easier. However, as will be discussed in Chapter 6, there are overwhelming advantages for many children in being educated in mainstream school. The limited social contact between teachers and SLTs as a regular feature of working life is fairly inevitable.

In lieu of the informal social interaction that comes from simply spending time working in the same setting, some services have produced documents that specify the functions and goals of the service, and the roles of the relevant professions in implementing these goals. Schools have made considerable progress by writing tailored policy documents concerning their approaches to special needs and support for learning. Many SLT services have produced similar documents, although these are probably less universal. Such documents can help to explain and clarify roles, responsibilities and expectations. This can defuse prior assumptions and prevent misunderstandings, and so make SLT visits to schools more comfortable.

Some of the problems can arise in sharing such documents, and in conveying the essence of the service to those outside the immediate professional readership. There is a need to do this, and to have easy dissemination of information.

Sharing information

An example worked through by Honeyfield (1997a) shows an attempt to deal with confusions surrounding an outreach service based in mainstream schools. Her post was as SLT attached to an outreach system which supported the integration into mainstream schools of children who attended, or who had previously attended, a part-time language unit. In this system, either a language support teacher or a language support SLT visited the child's mainstream school or nursery to work on previously contracted aims and objectives, usually within a small group in the classroom. At the same time, the school could be visited independently by other SLTs seeing children who were not associated with the language unit, and indeed staffing practicalities sometimes meant further complications. The system was carefully structured, but required to be explained to large numbers of staff, including headteachers, class teachers and secretaries across a number of schools, as well as to parents of children receiving the varieties of service provided.

The solution was to produce a one-page leaflet that could be liberally distributed and that listed and answered frequent and typical questions. These included:

- What is the language support team?
- What is outreach?
- Who will visit?
- What will they do?
- Is this 'speech therapy'?

Giving information in this way saved explanation time, and allowed a permanent record of the outreach system to remain in the hands of those who used the service, via the leaflet. It also showed the service in its overall organisational context, and 'legitimised' the presence of the SLT or support teacher in the classroom. Honeyfield (1997a) notes that parents expressed less anxiety about the transition from language unit to full-time school, and one mother said it was the first time she had realised 'it wasn't just a speech therapy group' her daughter had been attending. Headteachers reported that it was useful to have the leaflet to store with children's records, and class teachers found it useful to have information in the classroom to refer to if questioned by parents or to show to supply teachers or job-share partners.

Honeyfield (1997a, Appendix 1, pp 3-4)

Such small-scale, practical solutions are not trivial, and can make a large difference in developing good working relations. Documents do not replicate good social interaction, but by helping to explain a complex working context they may serve to foster mutual understanding and support.

Structural Issues

Structures describe the formalised ways in which services interact, and the prescribed arrangements for relating internally and to other services. The most obvious ways in which structures have been adapted to meet the needs of children with language and communication difficulties and to allow collaboration is in the setting-up of specialist schools and language units, and in the establishment of specialist SLT teams to work in such settings. MacKay and Anderson in Chapter 4 detail the rationale for setting up such units in one area, and comment on how they are operating. This chapter will give a more general overview, picking up issues identified in the previous chapter as affecting collaboration.

Timing and location of service delivery

The most obvious way in which difficulties in timing and location of service delivery have been reduced is by SLTs moving their services into schools, and indeed into classrooms, to foster collaboration. This removes some flexibility from the SLT service, and has caused some difficulties for SLTs in maintaining extensive contact with parents (Reid et al., 1996: 77). There are also problems to be overcome in introducing less experienced SLTs, such as newly qualified therapists, and student therapists into this situation (David and Smith, 1987; Roux, 1996). However, there have been obvious benefits in SLTs moving into schools, making collaboration with teachers much easier to implement.

The amount of time therapists work in classrooms varies across services. HMI in Scotland found many classroom-based examples; but also settings where the 'extract' model was the normal means of working, where the SLT chose to work almost exclusively in a separate room or where teachers virtually excluded therapists from the class. This clearly limited the amount of collaboration that could go on. Reid et al. (1996: 94) asked SLTs to list the occasions when extracting children would be the preferred form of service delivery, and the consensus was that extracting children was preferred on certain occasions: where the child had poor attention or the aims of the task would be relevant to one child only; where the child was using equipment that would be distracting to other children; when the problem was dysfluency (but see Lees in Chapter 7); and where a child, perhaps an older child, requested privacy. This would reinforce the need for a mix of locations for therapy to take place, but leave considerable opportunity for teachers and therapists to observe one another and work together in classrooms.

In the UK it is more common for teachers and SLTs to work together in the classroom in special schools and language units than in mainstream settings (Millar and Reid, 1996). In the USA, however, the move to integrate children with special educational needs into mainstream classes has to some extent been followed by therapy services also moving into classrooms. Structural and organisational features are different in that the USA has a cohort of school-based SLTs, employed by school services, who may not all have full SLT certification – but there are interesting parallels to be drawn.

Elksnin and Capilouto (1994) asked SLTs working mainly with young children in one US school district what they considered to be the advantages of working in the classroom, and what models of joint working they preferred and adopted. Beck and Dennis (1997) followed up this work, surveying teachers and SLTs using classroom-based interventions across two states. Respondents to both surveys felt that classroom-based work helped children to carry over language skills to real-life contexts, and kept children in their most natural environment, providing greater opportunities for appropriate reinforcement of classroom behaviours. Difficulties included finding joint planning time, discussed below, and at times targeting specific speech or language goals, reflecting perhaps the SLTs' concern with language forms as well as language use. Respondents to both surveys felt that 'team teaching', where both the SLT and the teacher presented the task to all children, was the best model of joint working, but both groups actually used the model 'one teach, one drift' (where one team member has primary responsibility for instruction and the other assists children with their work) more frequently. This may reflect the restrictions on planning time, as team teaching requires joint planning of sessions and activities, and respondents reported that such time was limited.

The US experience suggests that classroom-based service delivery can be successful, although the overall organisational context is different, and worries, barriers and tensions still exist. There can be difficulties in grouping children, and there remains a need for one-to-one interaction for severely disabled and developmentally young children (as discussed in a UK context by MacDonald and Rendle, 1994). However, those who adopted a model involving collaborating in a classroom felt that the reality of working in a rich learning environment offered ample compensation for any such difficulties.

Wherever work with children takes place, SLTs and teachers need time together to plan their actions, and finding time together can prove to be difficult. The lack of joint planning time is a recurring problem preventing good collaboration. Some organisation of services to allow shared planning time is necessary, and the following example illustrates the problems. Such examples suggest creative approaches, but also illustrate the serious resource limitations that militate against developing collaborative practice. The need to find more shared planning time continues to exercise service planners.

Finding planning time

Taylor (1997), as an SLT, needed to find time to discuss with teachers in a cooperative but heavily timetabled mainstream primary school. She ran up against the real difficulty of teachers having full class timetables with no cover available. Her post allowed her to be in the school on only one day a week, and there was a large caseload from up to six different classes. The teachers and SLT were unhappy with this lack of liaison time, but since teachers were unable to leave their classes discussion was mainly in classrooms with other children present, or at breaks.

After consultation, the headteacher and SLT agreed that the SLT would stop her contact with children at 2.45 pm and liaise with Primary 1 to Primary 3 teaching staff until 3.15 pm. If there were children in the upper stages of school, she would then liaise with their teachers from 3.15 pm onwards. At the start of Term 1 there would be an initial 20-minute discussion with each teacher who had a child receiving therapy, to allow joint planning and to set targets in each child's IEP. Since six teachers were involved, the short time available meant that these initial meetings could take up to 3 weeks to complete. The 10 minutes per teacher weekly discussion time after that would enable the evaluation of short-term targets and the planning of future targets.

The team found it helpful to have such a formal arrangement, and although the time allocation was still limited it proved more productive than informal arrangements. Joint planning in the curriculum improved. However, the time available was still barely adequate, and served as a limit to further collaboration.

Management structures

As outlined in Chapter 2, an inherent barrier to collaboration within management structures concerns the relative isolation of individual SLTs in the education context. This difficulty has been addressed in SLT services, both by developing overt team and trust-wide policy statements, and by adopting the RCSLT's professional standards as quoted above. These have helped to formulate good policy, and to contribute to the functional goals of service delivery, by giving individual SLTs frameworks for practice in the absence of elaborated on-site management structures.

However, another formal set of documents has proved useful in structuring collaborative working between schools and SLT services – the school-based service level agreement (Reid et al., 1996: 108). This spells out in considerable detail the amount of SLT service that a school will receive, and when it will be offered. It might also set out which parts of a child's programme will be delivered jointly in the classroom, and the quantity of teacher and SLT liaison time and when this will be timetabled. The amount and type of inservice training of teachers (by SLTs) and of SLTs (by teachers) can be listed, and the content and objectives of such training. Although this may seem a cumbersome and rather formal arrangement, the construction of such a document allows a school and SLT service to negotiate what they want from one another, and what the roles and responsibilities of each service will be. This can take a lot of the pressure away from individual SLTs and teachers, giving them a framework of expectations in which to establish collaborative practice. Reid et al. (1996) note that the potential for misunderstandings can be reduced, and that the agreement provides a basis for monitoring and evaluating provision.

School-based service-level agreements

Haggarty (1997) gives a useful personal account of procedures leading towards the writing of a service-level agreement which will be used to illustrate the process. As an SLT with extensive expertise in autism, she was responsible for setting up an SLT service in a newly established mainstream unit for young people on the autistic continuum. At the start of the process, both she and the experienced unit headteacher expected a collaborative approach, and were committed to its effectiveness.

After discussion, the following list of procedures was agreed on:

- The SLT would undertake inservice training with the teaching staff to outline her role, and explain how the service would operate.
- The SLT would work in the classroom setting alongside the teachers and auxiliaries.
- The SLT would attend specified meetings, or provide a report if she could not attend.
- Reports would be written by the SLT in conjunction with each pupil's review, and would form part of the unit's profile report..
- The class teacher, unit teacher and SLT would meet together on a regular basis to formulate the IEP for each pupil.
- Where possible, class teachers would be released from class for joint planning with the SLT.
- The unit head would devote a staff meeting once a month for staff to liaise with the SLT.
- The SLT would contribute to the unit's inservice programme.
- The SLT would inform the unit head in advance if she had to be away from the unit during her normal attendance time for any reason.

Discussion also took place on contact with parents, and on the importance of the SLT being involved across curriculum areas. Although the service-level agreement 'list' was useful in organising services, much further discussion and team building has been undertaken to develop the processes of collaboration.

Such a list might include features of interest to many schools and SLT services, although individual partnerships might want to emphasise different aspects of the list, to add to it or to omit some functions. Many would want to put amounts of time or frequency of meetings against points on the list. Choices will often be necessary, as the total package may have to be costed and come within a total amount of SLT time or resource allocated to the school. The advantage of such an agreement at school level is that roles and collaborative action can be planned for, evaluated and reviewed, taking individual realities into account.

Curriculum structures

Chapter 2 discussed the fact that the notion of a curriculum is somewhat alien in health service terms, but conversely that the very fact of concentrating on children's listening and talking abilities has given a proper focus to communication in education settings. As has happened with similar tensions over timing and location of service delivery, collaboration in the curriculum has been achieved by SLTs accepting the need to work in the national frameworks and to talk about children's language goals in ways that fit curriculum aims, as teachers do. The need to consider developmentally relevant aims and the inclusion of work on language forms has not been lost, but has rather been dealt with by differentiating in the curriculum, using the key strategies of individualisation, adaptation, enhancement and elaboration. Curriculum structures are now the normal mechanism for discussing children's learning in collaborative approaches.

The process of adapting the curriculum to individual children's needs requires considerable effort, however. Mason (1994) describes problems in matching the abilities of six children with speech and language disorders to the first level of the Scottish 5–14 Curriculum. She notes that expectations for attainment targets in the different curriculum strands vary, with the listening and talking strands being at a much simpler level than the reading and writing strands, and that there are no frameworks to encompass the actual difficulties in speech and language forms shown by the children. To make a curriculum approach possible, she had to write additional, developmentally sequenced steps leading up to the curriculum descriptor. Such adaptations are routinely required. A further example from practice appears below.

Writing curricular aims

Honeyfield (1997b), an SLT, was working with J, a 6-year-old child attending a mainstream school who had pragmatic difficulties in listening and conversation but good speech and syntactic development. As the Scottish 5–14 curriculum, like the English and Welsh national curriculum, is based on aspects of language use, it could be adapted fairly easily to meet his difficulties in attending and responding to stories and questions, and to maintaining a conversational topic.

This gave the following curricular aims:

1 **Working towards the listening strand – 'Listening for information, instructions and directions'**

   J will learn how to listen in a variety of situations.

J will learn the rules of sitting still, looking at the teacher and thinking about the words, first separately then all three together in the following situations:

– small group with SLT within class
– small group with class teacher within class
– larger group with class teacher and SLT within class
– whole class with SLT in class
– whole class with SLT at music/gym.

A variety of other children and activities will then be introduced in each situation.

2 Working towards the listening strand – 'Listening in groups'

(a) J will learn how to take turns talking and listening to group members.

J will learn the rules and vocabulary of turn-taking.
Teacher and SLT will use the vocabulary and state explicitly whose turn it is and what this means, e.g. 'It's Rob's turn to read, so everyone else look at him and think about the words'.

Groups and situations will progress as in Stage 1 above.

(b) J will understand, use and respond to 'ask' and 'tell':

J will learn the vocabulary 'ask' and 'tell'
J will be able to ask a question in a structured situation
J will be able to give an instruction in a structured situation
J will identify whether he was asked or told
J will be able to rephrase from request to command or vice versa.

3 Working towards the talking strand – 'Conveying information, instructions and directions'

J will give more information on request.

In small groups, J will give short descriptions or instructions to others.

J will think of more information in response to 'Tell me more' or 'Tell me something else'.

These aims were derived from detailed and repeated taping and pragmatic analysis of J's conversation by the SLT, and progress was evaluated in the same way. The aims were then fitted into the curriculum strands. The result allowed good collaboration between the teacher and SLT, through having a common terminology and through a closer fit between J's aims and the rest of the class work. The curriculum itself was not very helpful in suggesting these differentiated targets, and it was necessary to discuss how adaptations could be made.

Honeyfield (1997b, Appendix 1, pp 3-4)

Process Issues

Opening a statement or record of special education needs

Chapter 2 noted that there was considerable individual and local variation around decisions as to whether or not to open a statement or record of special educational needs, but no fundamental disagreement between SLT and education services about the underlying principles of doing this, which document and agree action on a child's education programme and curriculum adaptations. Difficulties and barriers tend to surface in two circumstances – when a special educational needs tribunal finds in favour of a form or level of service delivery that conflicts with the advice supplied by the local SLT service, and where there is a discrepancy between the stated needs of a child and available SLT provision. Solving either problem in favour of supplying SLT service to an individual child may give rise to inequalities in relation to other children, and indeed children with difficulties but without a statement or record of special education needs must also be assured of access to SLT services and have a fair share of resources directed to them.

These difficulties remain, but there has been further clarification of SLT collaboration in setting up a statement or record of needs and implementing its actions, in the form of principles and guidelines issued by the RCSLT (1997). These concern the role of the SLT in the cross-professional assessment of children with special needs, and dovetail with education procedures. IEPs should spell out the nature and type of advice that SLTs might helpfully offer, and the uses to which such advice may be put. This is a useful addition to the detailed work carried out by education services, and will help the process of setting up statements or records of special education needs for children with speech, language and communication disorders.

Planning for special needs

In planning for special needs, some good collaborative work takes place around the construction, implementation and development of children's IEPs, which map out the processes through which the system will organise a child's learning experiences. The construction of IEPs is advocated by both the code of practice (DfE, 1994, 1999) and the EPSEN document (SOEID, 1994), and involves writing aims for each child within the curriculum. They also provide a thorough framework within which to plan for a child's differentiated curriculum. HMI (1996: 24) gives a list of functions which should be served by an IEP.

'Best practice' IEPs
IEPs should:

- describe targets relating to pupils' language needs through setting out short-term (weekly), medium-term (3-monthly or termly) and long-term (school session) targets
- set out targets in the curriculum areas of English language, mathematics, and personal and social education and indicate how these are worked out throughout the whole curriculum
- describe resources and teaching strategies for meeting targets
- involve parents, teachers, educational psychologists, and occupational and speech and language therapists in jointly planning and evaluating the achievement of medium- and long-term targets
- involve speech and language therapists and teachers in jointly planning and evaluating the achievement of short-term targets
- pay due regard to pupils' wishes and maximise their involvement in setting and monitoring targets
- fulfil the requirements of pupils' statements or records of needs.

HMI (1996: 24)

IEPs, then, serve as a mechanism for integrating system processes. MacKinnon (1997) provides a practical example of developing and applying a collaborative framework in a language unit, within which the IEP plays an important and established part.

Setting IEPs

The unit served the needs of children with significant language disorder who had the cognitive potential to benefit from the mainstream curriculum. The children had independent self-care skills, and appropriate behaviour levels to allow supported integration into mainstream settings. The teaching and SLT staff were committed to joint goal setting, joint training, and monitoring and evaluation of working practices. Formal inservice and informal discussion sessions had covered the development and impairment of language, the structure and balance of the curriculum, and the interaction between the two in areas such as phonological awareness. Teacher and SLT contact was timetabled and therapists worked in classrooms, withdrawing children for individual work as required, for example for assessment. In addition, the assistant headteacher, educational psychologist and SLT met regularly to develop and evaluate policies, and the SLT manager monitored and reviewed service with the assistant headteacher. Home visits, parents' evenings, and a parents' support group, were arranged.

Joint teacher and SLT observation sheets covering language and literacy skills were developed and used in assessment, and IEPs were prepared.

IEPs contained information on:

- the members of the team responsible for the IEP
- a profile of the child's skills
- joint general aims and specific 5–14 curriculum aims
- weekly plans

- notes on the evaluation of progress
- a child self-review where possible.

The following sample IEP is from Steven, a 5-year-old boy with a pre-school history of speech and language difficulty who met the unit's entry criteria. Steven's pupil profile showed:

- he had some verbal comprehension problems, but understood situations and routines. Formal assessment showed a significant verbal comprehension impairment
- he used single nouns but only one two-word phrase ('X's turn'). Intelligibility was poor because of limited speech sound development. He used some gesture
- visual perception and visual memory were areas of strength
- he had fairly poor gross-motor skills (i.e. he could not hop) but good fine-motor skills
- he tended to be isolated in play situations and had independent self-care routines
- he was good at puzzles and could match and sort shapes, colours and sizes
- he had a number of strengths to offset his specific language impairment.

General aims were agreed for inclusion in the IEP:

1 To improve communication effectiveness with the introduction of a simple signing system for use in class and at home.
2 To increase the range and amount of expressive language used in conjunction with the above.
3 To improve comprehension of language including introduction of new vocabulary and also length of instruction understood.
4 To improve auditory skills including auditory sequential memory and listening skills.

With these aims in mind, an IEP was drawn up, as follows:

Curriculum strand – listening

Listening for information, instructions and directions

Targets	Develop comprehension up to three information carrying word level
Activities	Derbyshire Language Scheme (Knowles and Masidlover, 1982)
Personnel	SLT

Listening in groups

Targets	Improve ability to listen without distraction in group
Activities	AFASIC 'Activities for listening' (Anderson et al., 1990) Music box, taped listening games
Personnel	Classroom assistant

Curriculum strand – talking

Conveying information, instructions and directions

Targets	Use of augmentative communication system
Activities	Makaton (Walker, 1976)
Personnel	Team, including parents, taxi staff, dinner staff SLT to arrange inservice

Targets	Increase range of words used, e.g. verbs and adverbs
Activities	Derbyshire Language Scheme, Makaton, Let's Play Language (Barnett and Fletcher-Wood, 1983)
Personnel	SLT, class teacher, classroom assistant

Curriculum strand – reading

Reading for information

Targets	Identify and interpret sight vocabulary in different contexts
Activities	Oxford Reading Tree (OUP, 1986)
Personnel	Class teacher

Curriculum strand – writing

Personal

Targets	Drawing action pictures of self
Activities	Foundations of Writing (Michael and Michael, 1987)
Personnel	Class teacher, classroom assistant

Spelling

Targets	Awareness of rhyme
Activities	'Each Peach Pear Plum' Topic (Burnell and Harkness, 1992)
Personnel	SLT, class teacher

Curriculum strand – information handling

Interpretation

Targets	Sort and count by shape and size
Activities	HI Note Book, Derbyshire Language Scheme
Personnel	Class teacher, SLT

Curriculum strand – money, measurement, number

Range and type of numbers

Targets	Number ordering to 10
Activities	HI Books, Compare Bears (Hewett 1986)
Personnel	Class teacher

Measuring

Targets	Understanding big, small
Activities	Compare Bears
Personnel	Class teacher, SLT

At a weekly evaluation and planning time, key personnel fed back on Steven's progress. The plan for the following week was agreed and the long-term aims modified if appropriate, with one team member leading the discussion, taking notes and circulating the relevant paperwork.

This planning mechanism worked well in the unit setting, although it would have been difficult to run in other settings, such as the mainstream, as the practical difficulties in arranging planning and evaluation time could have been too great. There was a trade-off for SLTs between such an integrated approach and individual, one-to-one contact with the children, which required a shift in focus to see therapy as supporting and enabling the child to cope with the demands of education by integrating 'therapy' and curricular work.

MacKinnon (1997)

IEPs have great benefits for joint planning, and serve as a focus at the process level for ensuring that individual children receive and benefit from collaborative approaches. A further detailed example is given in Chapter 5 by Mackay and Young.

Systems Environment

The systems environment in which services operate consists of those who have a stake in the system and interests in it. There is a reciprocal interaction between services and their systems environment, each impinging on the other.

Families of children receiving services are an obvious example of stakeholders, as are children themselves, whose interests and rights have been strengthened by the Children Act (1989–91 and 1995–7, Scotland). McCool in Chapter 8 gives a detailed account of models of working with parents, and a worked example of how one school tries to accommodate parents' perspectives with those of professionals. As well as parents and carers themselves, parents' organisations and support services such as AFASIC and IPSEA publish policy, good practice and information packs which can be useful in providing frameworks against which services can test their own actions.

In Scotland, a policy-making and professional advice-giving service is provided by the strongly influential HMI, whereas in England and Wales Ofsted carries out an inspection role that can lead to policy suggestions. In the health service, professional bodies such as the RCSLT help in policy making and establishing good practice, as well as organisations concerned with policy studies such as the King's Fund. Below the national levels of influence there are also LEA and NHS trust level policies, and local community interests that affect practice in both school and SLT services.

Apart from parents, the above mentioned bodies have statutory ways of influencing services, or collect resources to allow them to publicise and disseminate their opinions. Parents are, however, a special case and warrant further discussion.

Families and services

Chapter 2 noted the tensions that can exist between families' and schools' expectations of how SLT services would be delivered, and Chapter 1 mentioned how the law concerning statements and records of special educational needs was influenced by parents who were not satisfied when the amount of SLT provision received by their child fell short of expectation.

Ways of dealing with such tensions have mostly centred around explanations and information giving, such as Honeyfield's (1997a) example above, and McCool in Chapter 8 also gives an example of adaptations to reporting mechanisms that helped to explain the functions and processes of a service. However, as noted in Chapter 2, Reid et al. (1996: 102) found few examples of parents being actively involved in setting goals and planning curriculum adaptations for children. None the less, Reid et al. (1996) also noted that more than three-quarters of the parents they interviewed felt adequately included in decisions about their child's overall needs and difficulties. This appears to indicate a general level of parental satisfaction, but there is room for much more parental involvement. Parents can be generally happy with services while making comparison with other experiences and still requiring further information and reassurance. McCaughey (1997b) caught some of the issues concerning parents' experiences in both a medical and education model in an interview with parents, Mr and Mrs C, whose son of 5 years and 9 months had recently moved to a language unit.

Parents' involvement in two services

The family had received services for their child from a child development centre (CDC) for a year, and C had recently received a part-time placement at a local language development unit (LDU) attached to a primary school. He continued to attend the CDC for services other than SLT.

McCaughey had been C's SLT in the CDC, and had been appointed to the LDU at the same time as C began attendance there. She therefore had a good relationship with Mr and Mrs C, and personal knowledge of the workings of both the CDC and the LDU. As she had been the SLT in both settings, there were unlikely to be issues arising from a change of therapy style or personnel which influenced parents. Mr and Mrs C agreed to be interviewed by her at home, to discuss their perceptions of both services. A rough agenda for the meeting was supplied the day before.

The CDC used a multidisciplinary model with a strong commitment to family support. The LDU was also committed to families, but parental contact was limited by the fact that children came from a fairly wide geographical area and (unlike the CDC) there was no transport provided for parents, although public transport links were good.

The parents' pertinent comments were:

Location, transport and travel
'I couldn't guarantee my attendance at CDC appointments without the support of the transport services.'

'The unit is out of bounds to me, because of where it is, and prevents me from attending the monthly parents' group meeting.'

Access to staff
Initially, Mrs C found the CDC team 'too big' and she was afraid they would 'take over'. Over time she realised that they 'listened to my opinions' and the continuity of seeing the same professionals, particularly the doctor, helped her build good relationships and feel more confident.

On her first visit to the LDU Mrs C was aware that the staff had an immediate understanding of C's difficulties. However, as he was escorted to and from the LDU, 'I can't talk to the staff face to face' and 'telephoning to ask for a progress report imposes on the staff's time'.

'The home/school diary is a timetable of C's morning, and tells us nothing about his performance in the unit.' By contrast, 'After C's sessions at the CDC I get to hear about what he's been doing and how well he's done, but I don't get that kind of information from the unit'.

On reports
The CDC sent copies of the various therapists' reports but not the doctor's report to parents, and gave a verbal report at the end of each session. Parents said, 'We don't need a copy of the doctor's report as I'm in on the session and I know how well [C] has done anyway'.

The LDU provided written reports before review meetings, and the parents approved – 'We like getting the LDU report before the meeting, as then we know there will be no surprises on the day'.

On case review meetings
'Some of the [CDC] meetings were too big, and it was hard for me to say my piece.'

The parents were happy that all professionals at the LDU meeting reached the same conclusions about C as the parents, and that their opinions had been valued.

General suggestions
Mr and Mrs C thought that the following general points should be thought about:

- When children are initially accepted into the unit, time should be set aside to explain the principles of the service to parents, to reduce confusion at a later date.
- Parents need clearer information about the collaborative approach teachers and SLTs take to the preparation and planning of integrated activities. This will reduce the anxieties parents have about therapy time versus teaching time.
- The communication system between the unit and parents needs clarification.
- The problem of the location of the unit for parents has to be acknowledged, and the possibility of home visits for parents needs to be looked at.

McCaughey (1997: 1-7)

This interview captures many of the issues raised by parents as they move among systems and settings. Good collaborative practice will develop as issues such as those C's parents express are routinely raised and addressed, with parents included in a thoroughgoing way.

The Systems Implications

SLT services and teachers are working together, and evidence for this has been presented at all levels of the systems model. To a large extent, this is because SLTs have adopted schools' perspectives, and tried to fit their services into an education context, while adapting certain aspects. Examples of this are the SLTs' willingness to use the language of the curriculum, and to work in classroom contexts. However, the model remains one of collaboration and not assimilation, and SLT perspectives have remained in independent policy statements, clarification of roles and individualised curriculum activities reflecting SLTs' areas of expertise. This suggests that good collaborative practice can continue to develop and that SLT–teacher partnerships can continue to be productive.

Chapter 4
Specialist Services for Pupils with Disorders of Language and Communication: Policies, Practice and Perceptions

GILBERT MacKAY AND CAROLYN ANDERSON

Introduction

This chapter will consider collaboration between SLTs and teachers with reference to a 1997 study in the west of Scotland of services for children described as having 'disorders of language and communication'. This area may not be typical of the whole of the UK, but a thorough analysis of a limited geographical area will allow discussion of issues concerning policies, practice and perceptions that will have relevance to the broader issues of setting up specialist services for children with language and communication difficulties.

The study (originally reported in MacKay et al., 1997) was carried out because of pressure on the authors' departments for postgraduate education for teachers and SLTs. These demands had resulted directly from a proliferation of education authority provision for children with disorders of language and communication. Such proliferation was part of a broader movement for the development of specialist recognition and provision in Scotland in an area that had received little attention since the Education (Scotland) Act (1945). Subsequent 1954 'Regulations' (equivalent to those of 1959 in England and Wales) designated 'speech defect' as a possible source of difficulties in learning. The area had remained something of a Cinderella with respect to the provision of specific facilities and interest until the production of a report, 'Children with Communication Disorders', by the principal psychologists of the Scottish education authorities in 1988 (Working Party of Scottish Principal Educational Psychologists, 1988). (Chapter 1 gives an overall account of the development of services for children with language and communication difficulties.) From 1991, a combination of parental pressure on parliament and activity by HMI gave it further prominence. Since then, there has been an expansion in provision and in interest at rates unsurpassed in the previous four decades, and this growth is not complete. It is reasonable to say that those with personal and professional interests in this specialism were pleased to see its rise in priority for attention. Yet, such attention should also be seen in the broader context of the nature and dynamics of a changing system.

In the geographical area where the research was carried out, there had been a powerful movement against the development of services with a specialised focus. Autism and dyslexia are examples of such specialisms. Even recognising the more encompassing term 'disorders of language and communication' ran counter to a prevailing trend of providing for the special needs of pupils with low-incidence disorders through generic 'learning support' – a system designed to meet the needs of the almost indefinable group of pupils described as having 'learning difficulties'. Some of the thinking behind this approach is outlined in Chapter 2, when discussing functional issues of education provision versus 'deficit' models of practice. Here it will be helpful to fill in some more of the background in Scottish learning support, as it has had such an important influence on policy and practice in education authorities.

Learning support

The learning support movement drew its momentum from a Scottish Office document (contemporary with the Warnock Report) that recommended radical overhaul of thinking and practices in what was then called 'remedial education' (HMI, 1978). Learning support acquired a particularly clear function from the early 1990s when the National Curriculum (England and Wales) and the 5–14 Curriculum (Scotland) emerged as the frameworks in which education in state schools should be set. Its function is to help pupils who have difficulty in learning to achieve targets in these frameworks. Without question, learning support should take credit for changing attitudes and practices: teachers and pupils no longer see the provision of specialist support as something that is delivered by remedial teachers in separate bases. Instead, pupils usually receive assistance in their own classes, and giving that assistance can be as much the responsibility of their class teachers as of the learning support staff. Spreading responsibility for support has also helped to broaden and clarify the definition of special educational needs. Soon after 1978, there was much discussion of Warnock's estimate that 20% of pupils had special education needs, not just the 1–2% who might have their education in special schools. That debate is largely a thing of the past: it is widely assumed that anyone may require support at some time in his or her school career. Special support is not only for the few.

Learning support is undoubtedly responsible for the development of worthy attitudes and practice in Scottish schools, but it has a troublesome converse message that has been broadcast particularly by inservice courses in teacher-education institutions throughout the 1990s. The message is that barriers to learning exist solely in the pupil's environment, not in the individual's personal characteristics. Thus, hearing impairment, autism or cerebral palsy are not barriers to learning because they are within the pupil. This position can be interesting as a focus for debate, as Tobin (1998) has recently demonstrated with reference to blindness, but it has practical consequences when it becomes a basis for action. For example, there is widespread belief in the region where the study took place that generic forms of learning support are the appropriate forms of special provision for virtually all pupils. By contrast, support designed for pupils with specific types of disability, and even specialised knowledge of specific disabilities, is often dismissed as reflecting 'medical' and 'deficit' models of thinking, a theme discussed elsewhere in this chapter and in Chapter 2.

This was the context in which a rapid and, it appears, reactive and loosely planned proliferation of language units to provide a new specialist support service for pupils with disorders of language and communication began in Scotland around 1991. The study reported in this chapter outlines the development of this new service, and draws attention to a number of matters of principle and practice that need to be resolved, and that are pertinent to provision across the UK. Their relevance can often be highlighted by reference to the development of Banathy's (1992) systems approach (McCartney et al., 1998) cited throughout this volume. The systems approach will indicate problems of definition and interpretation which must be addressed by education and health authorities, and also by voluntary agencies and pressure groups. Solutions may not be comfortable because, on the one hand, they challenge the rhetoric of the prevailing context in the field of special education with its restricted view of the ways in which children's needs may be understood. Yet, on the other hand, they also challenge the voluntary sector, which is enjoying attention because of the apparent clarity and accessibility of vision that comes from having the simplistic goal of more provision of services.

Context

The upsurge of interest in pupils with disorders of language and communication led the Scottish Office to sponsor three studies in this area, which are mentioned throughout this book. First, HMI undertook a study of schools and units for children with disorders of language and communication, and produced a report that is essential reading (HMI, 1996). In association with that study, two reviews of the field (Donaldson, 1995; Trevarthen et al., 1996) were commissioned and published. Second, a team from the University of Edinburgh and Queen Margaret College (Reid et al., 1996) reviewed the role of SLTs in relation to pupils with special educational needs (SEN). The SLTs' role seems critical in providing specialist education for pupils with disorders of language and communication, but it is not developed extensively in the report of Reid et al. (1996) because of their concern with different issues relating to collaborative working between the fields of health and education. Third, Jordan and Jones reported their findings on provision for pupils with autism in June 1997.

There is considerable diversity of services, both in existence and in preparation, among Scottish education authorities. It was important to investigate this diversity to contribute knowledge that might help in policy building, decision taking and in creating networks of shared interest among practitioners and administrators. The following areas of inquiry emerged as key issues to examine in the west of Scotland in evidence drawn from HMI (1996) and from information given by four cohorts of teachers and one of SLTs on specialist postgraduate courses.

Area 1: types of provision offered

The range of provision for children with language and communication difficulties was diverse. What was it? What types of provision appeared most frequently, and what gaps in provision appeared to exist?

Area 2: identification of pupils and definition of their difficulties

Practitioners often appeared unsure of the specific remits of individual units. For example, unit A is described as a 'language unit'. May it admit children with autistic difficulties? Such confusion seemed to have three roots. First was the rapidity with which new units emerged in the years from 1990: there had been virtually no previous service with which to compare them. Whom, then, were they supposed to serve? Second was the problem of making a reliable classification of the difficulties presented by children. Third was the resistance by special needs administrators in the region's former education authority to use of the term 'autism': 'communication disorder' became the required nomenclature for 'autism' and 'Asperger syndrome'. Thus, the study aimed to discover the extent to which terminology was an important issue in the development and provision of services.

Area 3: staffing and management of the services

The widespread provision for children with disorders of language and communication is a relatively new phenomenon, and had not been addressed by Scottish teacher-education institutions as an area for professional development until recently. What were the backgrounds of the staff of the services, and what procedures existed to facilitate children's progress towards, through and beyond the services?

The Project

An interview schedule, based on the three areas outlined above, was drawn up, for administration in the 12 new councils that emerged from the former Strathclyde region in the local government reorganisation of 1996. Interviews were carried out in only 11 of these, as one authority made no specific provision for pupils with disorders of language and communication at the time of the study. In general, the study's respondents were officials such as education officers, principal officers (SEN and learning support), advisers and principal psychologists. All were sent copies of the schedule in advance of an individual interview.

Two interviews were carried out by telephone, the remainder face to face. The authorities were willing participants in the study, and offered cooperation that went beyond the initial requirements of the project. For example, one education officer asked the researchers to make contact with the staff in his authority's specialist communication centre, to ensure a comprehensive gathering of information from those who delivered the service. Another asked one of the researchers to take part in an inservice day for teachers and SLTs; from this contact it was possible to have issues illuminated by those responsible for service delivery. Over the course of the study, additional information regularly came in informal exchanges with staff in schools, units and education administration.

Questions from the three original areas were useful as a means of eliciting information, but the balance of findings indicated a somewhat different range of priorities. These findings are now reported in a sequence that draws attention to the main issues that emerged.

Findings

Extent of provision

One difficulty encountered throughout the project was that of obtaining reliable quantitative data. On a number of occasions, situations were changing as data were being gathered, and this referred to matters as substantial as the number of services identified. It was possible to report that there was a total of 33 units in the authorities surveyed at Easter 1997: a breakdown of the forms they took appears in MacKay et al. (1997). Most existed in the form of units, attached either to mainstream schools or to offices of the psychological service. Two schools also existed, one for pupils of primary age with a variety of language disorders, the other for pupils from a wider age range with severe disorders that might be described more economically as 'autism'. The best estimate of the total number of pupils for whom these services made provision would be about 550–600 children, although a constantly changing situation made it difficult to give a reliable figure. Across the authorities, perhaps two in every thousand pupils were receiving support from a unit, service or school specialising in disorders of language and/or communication. That proportion must also be treated with caution because, as will be reported below, most pupils who received special provision were of primary or pre-school age. It is probably fair to conclude that the majority of primary-age pupils with disorders of language and communication either receive no special support designated specifically for their disorders, or receive it from more generic services such as learning support, behaviour support and special schools.

Various lines of reporting were encountered. Units located in premises of psychological services were usually the responsibility of these services. Those in primary schools were usually responsible to the headteacher of the school where they were located through an assistant headteacher who was head of the unit. However, the place of this line of reporting was not universal, nor was it necessarily likely to continue. For instance, some units were heading for a greater administrative detachment from their base schools, with line-reporting to an education officer rather than the headteacher. Conversely, one authority was moving towards more involvement of a unit's head in non-unit activities in the mainstream of the school. There was no homogeneity of staff-structures across the primary units surveyed. Most were under the direction of an assistant headteacher (as mentioned above), but at least one was directed by a non-promoted member of staff at the time of the survey.

The age of services varied considerably from that of pre-school and early education language units, which were at least 20 years old [founded around the publication of the Bullock Report – DES (1975)], to units that were on the point of opening in 1997. The period of rapid expansion in the establishment of services began with the deliberation of 1991, mentioned above, and continues.

The systems approaches of Banathy (1992) and McCartney et al. (1998) would suggest that the unresolved definition of structures across these services might be a source of difficulties. Arguably, problems with function and system-environment interaction (mentioned later) might be more important. However, an earlier study that used Banathy's systems approach found that poorly designed structures impaired the development of a service in virtually all areas of its functioning (MacKay et al., 1996).

Services provided

There were two commonly found types of provision for children of primary-school age and younger. The first was full-time day placement, with the intention that pupils would sooner or later transfer to a mainstream (or perhaps special) school in their home areas. That sort of provision typified units covering the whole primary-school range from 5 to 11 years. A second type of unit was found in some authorities for pupils aged from 3 years to 7–8 years (Primary 3). Such units tended to give half-day provision for children with delays or disorders of language. This second type of provision was common in the services that emerged around the time of the Bullock Report (DES, 1975), indicating how old is our faith in early intervention services that may begin too late.

Four less common types of provision should also be noted, of which the first were units in two mainstream secondary schools, under the direction of a principal teacher, responsible to the headteacher of the school. Their pupils showed greater or lesser degrees of autistic behaviour, although the severity of pupils' difficulties appeared to vary between the two. In one, a principal task of the unit was to give support to its four pupils and to teachers throughout the school so that the pupils might spend as much of their time as possible in mainstream classes. In the other unit, the pupils appeared to have greater degrees of difficulty and to spend most of their time in the unit itself. The staff tried to maintain some of the routines of standard secondary schooling: the pupils were in year groups – Secondary 1, 2 and 3 – and changed subjects at the end of periods.

Second, one school provided day and residential education for up to 24 pupils, covering the age range from 5 years to 16 years, and beyond. The school's handbook described the pupils as having 'severe language and communication disorders', the only term by which the previous education authority was prepared to recognise autism. Third, one primary school (which could accommodate 18 pupils) is probably the only school that has existed in Scotland for pupils with language disorders. Lastly, two councils provided units for pupils with phonological disorders.

Support through outreach and general learning support services

The outreach activities mentioned by the study's respondents were principally liaison between units and the mainstream schools from which pupils in primary-age units had come. Liaison occurred particularly in relation to shared placements and to the transition of pupils back to their local schools. There were relatively few reports of staff in communication services providing mainstream schools with the type of support that is given by specialist teachers of pupils with physical, visual and hearing impairments. However, there is evidence of willingness among teachers and SLTs to develop this type of service. Peripatetic practice appears to have been encountered more frequently by Reid et al. (1996: 9), and therefore findings in the area of Scotland covered by this study may not be representative of other areas of the UK.

The lack of such provision or specialism may be an effect of the relative recency of interest in this area, and the recency of the existence of specialist postgraduate courses. In addition, there was general agreement across the councils that staff working in general learning support services would be involved in the support of children with language and communication disorders. It is likely, indeed, that class teachers, SLTs and general learning support services are responsible for attending to the special needs of most pupils with disorders of language and communication as such small numbers receive attention from the specialist centres and schools: as stated above, possibly about two pupils in every thousand attended one of the specialist units or schools, and they were almost exclusively pupils of primary age. The services reviewed are in a state of unpredictable development; and the emergence of new services may influence the uptake of placements and the demand for them.

No respondent in the study expressed a need to have disorders of language and communication as a specialism in the mainstream learning support service, although there were some signs that such a specialism may emerge. This evidence is worth reading in the context of Reid et al. (1996: 9). They drew attention to the more effective collaborative working practices between teachers and SLTs that appeared in special rather than mainstream education facilities. They also recommended 'the creation of more places in special education facilities for pupils with significant speech, language and communication difficulties'.

Terminology

There was widespread acceptance across the councils of the prescribed terminology of the former Strathclyde region. The term 'communication disorder' was used almost exclusively to describe autism and related disorders. A few respondents did use the term 'autism' to describe the behaviour of children with these characteristics, and seemed comfortable with this. One respondent disliked the term and would not usually use it. Another stated explicitly that 'communication disorder' is used to describe 'the continuum of autism'. By contrast, 'disorders of language' was used to cover all other aspects of this field, including difficulties of delayed language, understanding of language and performance of speech acts. The following quotation was given by the only respondent in the study who attempted to define 'language' and 'communication' in terms different from the Strathclyde canon: '"Communication" has to do with support for the use of language, and "language" has to do with support for the development of speech and communication'.

The respondent defined communication disorder, therefore, as one area of pragmatic problems, and language delay and disorder as problems that impair the development or quality of communication. The respondent acknowledged the difficulties in maintaining a reliable distinction, a difficulty that is also recognised throughout the HMI report. However, he had moved to a functional way of understanding the difficulties from the more diagnostic labelling of equating disorders of communication to autistic disorders. That way of understanding has interesting parallels with the reluctance of many SLTs to use either modern or well-established classification categories because they believe that functional descriptions, and responses to the descriptions, offer more effective routes to delivering a service. Yet, Attwood (1998) makes a valid contrary case when he argues for the use of labels that will secure the best provision.

Staffing and size of services

Above, there have been references to the state of flux affecting many of the services, with its consequent difficulties for quantifying reliably the number of pupils being served. The issue here is less the number of children than the potential effects of the fluid situation. For example, one newly formed unit could say that its current roll was five pupils, but the imminent opening of a second class would raise this to about 10. However, it was possible that the unit might have to fulfil an 'assessment and throughput' function for at least several months because of council priorities, in which case the roll of long-term and short-term pupils would rise to 16. Even short-term planning is fraught with uncertainty in such circumstances, where processes and structures have to change unpredictably to accommodate new functions and areas of focus for the service.

In units attached to schools or psychological services, the ratio of teachers to pupils was about 1:5. Invariably, auxiliary staff were also available. No clear pattern emerged among the backgrounds of teachers who staffed the units and schools. Most were primary teachers originally, although a few came from physical education or secondary subjects. Data were not complete, but it would be fair to estimate that half had no accredited training in SEN, and half had either a diploma in SEN or support for learning. A small number held the advanced certificate in autism from Birmingham University.

SLTs were associated with all services, although the extent of their involvement varied from that of full-time placement to part-time consultancy. This issue is discussed by Reid et al. (1996) and relates to the administrative arrangements, which vary considerably across health boards and trusts. In our study, it seemed that the most effective collaboration took place when SLTs had a major part of their time allocated to the special services; where they and teachers could work in close proximity when this was appropriate; and where the individual therapists had autonomy over how best to use their time. This reflects the discussion in Chapter 3, and suggests once again that structure is an important component in collaboration.

Procedures

Referrals came from a variety of sources but the two most frequently mentioned routes to the admission panels of schools and units were psychological services and pre-school assessment teams.

Admission to provision and transfer from it were enabled by two processes. The first was the specification of criteria for potential referrers to the service, although problems with the reliability of criteria were reported, and are discussed below. The second process was the universal use of admission panels – teams consisting of teachers, SLTs and educational psychologists. Parents attended admissions meetings in about half of the services, and thereafter routinely attended review meetings of their children's progress. Professionals' pleas for the development of parent–service relationships have been heard since the principal psychologists' report (Working Party of Scottish Principal Educational Psychologists, 1988). Repeatedly, teachers and SLTs told us that it was essential to make time to listen to parents and to talk with them. On the one hand, parents' understanding of their children is critical, practical information, invaluable for developing professionals' awareness of needs, complex conditions and effective responses. On the other hand, respect for parents' understanding is essential if they are to have confidence in the services provided for their children. Further discussion of parents' roles is found in Chapter 8.

There was no definite pattern to determine the opening of records of needs (the Scottish 'statement') in the services surveyed. In general, the older the children or the more severe their disorders, the more likely were they to have records of needs.

Discussion

Terminological problems, including 'communication' and 'autism'

Continuing problems with terminology were evident. The 1954 'speech defect' is clearly out of date, but the current 'disorders of language and communication' is still far from satisfactory. A case can be made for advocating the use of 'disorders of communication' (the preference of the principal psychologists in 1988) as the generic term because effective language without communication is not much of an educational goal. It is essential that practitioners and policy makers should address the area of terminology because of the confusion that emanates from an apparent reluctance to identify and define the focus of these new services, and the environment to which they relate. The anti-labelling case is not difficult to grasp, and can be accommodated easily in systems that have clarified their functions and goals.

As reported earlier, only one respondent in the study defined a distinction between 'language' and 'communication'. All other respondents, if they made a distinction at all, reflected the reluctance of their former employer to use terms specifically naming autism and Asperger syndrome. Admittedly, there are problems of defining these terms too, but it is hard to defend the coyness that blankets autistic disorders under the label 'communication'. Using terms such as 'communication difficulties' to encompass all the range of autistic behaviour is neither accurate in reality nor just to the families affected by it. Conversely, it also suggests that pupils with difficulties in speech and language do not have a difficulty with effective communication. This is not the case.

Some confusion could be lifted by regarding all education provision for pupils with disorders of speech, language and communication as 'communication centres', because effective communication is a primary goal of all of the services surveyed. 'Social and communication disorders', used in some parts of Scotland, has a strong claim for attention too, for 'social' adds to the understanding of educational goals for children with pragmatic disorders and autistic behaviour. However, there is also a danger that 'social' may detract from a comprehensive understanding of the roots and phenomena of such behaviour. There is no strong reason to hang back from referring openly to autism when there are children whose behaviour may be described succinctly and appropriately by such terminology.

By contrast, there should also be recognition of the diversity of conditions in the autistic syndrome in the creation and development of services. Wing and Gould's (1979) 'triad of social impairments' may be a useful first framework of response: the ideas are already familiar to many practitioners, do not reduce autism to a simplistic 'disorder of communication', and provide a functional description of the presentation and effects of autistic behaviour. Yet, there is a danger that the triad may be a shibboleth that protects its users from scrutiny, or that [as Trevarthen et al. (1996: 11) indicate] it may inhibit the influence of more modern ideas on the importance of intrinsic motivation in communication.

In addition, the validity of the current popular metaphors of a 'spectrum' or 'continuum' of autism should be debated more openly because their use, and the contrasting disapproval of terms such as 'autistic tendency', is not an area where debate is encouraged by some guardians of autism's glossary. Informal evidence from the services shows that some teachers and SLTs have moved beyond the 'triad'. In particular, there were reports of staff's advances with approaches that respect pupils' idiosyncratic attempts to explore and communicate as an essential basis for learning. Straightforward functional analysis, too, has a place in enabling children to overcome their puzzling impairments. There are also reports of the value of techniques for assisting language development in children whose speech is already well advanced, but whose capacity to use it is not.

Identification of pupils

In terms of the systems framework referred to in other parts of this volume, there is a 'process' problem with respect to the placement of pupils in special services, and their transition from them to long-term education placement. Informal discussions with staff in the special services indicated concern and confusion about admissions criteria and about the influence of gatekeepers, particularly educational psychologists, who often had little specialist knowledge of this area of education. One sequel to the study has been a proposal for addressing the issue by an intuitive scaling approach (derived from MacKay and Lundie, 1998), in which each of a team of professionals is asked to use rating scales to assign 'fuzzy' numerical scores (see, for example, Fourali, 1997) to different aspects of children's communicative, social and education competence. The aim is to clarify the differing perceptions of an individual child that exist among the team, to assist in taking decisions about the meeting of children's needs. This work is in its early stages, and will be reported on in due course.

Secondary pupils

The special needs of pupils of secondary age are a matter of concern. It is undoubtedly the case that the needs of many children will change as they grow older. Some children may cease to have special needs, so that a response to them through the provision of a communication centre, or other type of earlier support, may not be appropriate. For example, many young children with disorders of communication or delays in language development will overcome these difficulties to the extent that mainstream education, with or without special support, is the only appropriate placement for them. Some with delayed language development may have difficulty as part of more global developmental difficulties which become the priority for response.

Yet, there will remain a proportion of pupils with persistent difficulties in communication that will remain with them always. In the course of the study, there were three references only to the support of secondary pupils, two concerning existing services and one to a service in preparation. This is an area for a more focused response to ensure that the special needs of secondary pupils are recognised and met. Such specificity of response may appear contrary to the non-categorising ethos of the 1981 Acts on both sides of the border. Yet, teachers cannot ignore an individual's specific difficulty on the one hand and, on the other, respond to the individuality of that person's needs for a broad and balanced curriculum. That dilemma is in the nature of teaching pupils who have special needs. In any case, it is possible that avoiding the naming of disabling conditions is a passing fashion: labels akin to those of the 1954 (Scottish) and 1959 (English and Welsh) regulations appear in 'Effective Provision for Special Education Needs' (SOEID, 1994: 41) and the code of practice for England and Wales (DfE, 1994). Avoidance of labels for its own sake can be avoidance of the reality of disability, with the consequent failure to recognise the rights to special provision that are stated in the UN Charter on the Rights of the Child.

Professional development

The study from which this chapter emerged had its roots in a need for more and better professional development. The study makes us believe that the investment of time in planning new courses has been justified. Such professional development is mainly available to teachers and SLTs through formal postgraduate courses but other types of opportunity also exist.

In the course of the study, one of the councils surveyed organised a staff development day in which a group of teachers and SLTs participated. All expressed a need for joint postgraduate training of experienced professionals. Teachers and SLTs may have different views of needs. Teachers are rightly concerned with access to a curriculum that is part of the normal process of enculturation. Therapists are rightly concerned with responding to difficulties. No model of response, such as 'curricular', 'developmental', 'individual', 'deficit', 'therapeutic' or 'medical' is right or wrong intrinsically – they are no more than ways of knowing, which may be appropriate in some circumstances, and not in others. Yet, there are also significant areas of overlap that must be recognised in professional practice. Staff attending the development day recognised the benefits of joint planning and operating. Interprofessional development events, involving staff from a large single service or from a group of smaller neighbouring services, could be organised with little effort. They should promote understanding of the legitimately different outlooks of education and therapy by focusing on the shared daily practice of the participants.

The existence of the differing but equally legitimate perspectives of teachers and SLTs draws attention to one of the deeper problems with contemporary service, and perhaps education services particularly, for people with special needs. In recent years, it has been fashionable to label any approach or service that responds to an identified disorder such as autism, hearing impairment or intellectual disability as a 'deficit' or 'medical' 'model'. Such rhetoric performed a useful function in the 1970s, when it was often important to advise caution against the assess-prescribe-treat model of practice that had been adopted enthusiastically because of the dramatic changes in people's lives that were often achieved by behaviour modification. That argument does not have the same relevance in the 1990s, because behaviour modification has itself undergone modification in the intervening years. The accusation of 'deficit' and 'medical' thinking seems now to be made if practitioners recognise disabilities as relevant sources of difficulty when identifying and responding to people's special needs. Of course, it is legitimate to understand children as elements in a system, such as school, home or community. But it is equally legitimate to understand them as individuals whose lives are affected by personal characteristics, including abilities and disabilities. Both forms of understanding are important in ensuring that the forms of service created to support their education take account of the whole individual. In the region studied, an exclusive way of understanding children with disabilities had become the 'official knowledge' (Apple, 1993) of learning support. Its reluctance to accept the reality of disabilities and their effects is a failure to recognise the totality of individuals, which may put at risk their chances of having an education service that meets their needs.

In systems terms, restricting perceptions of pupils and their needs to one way of knowing can obscure the 'function' and 'environment' of special services. In practical terms, as mentioned above, this has created difficulties for admissions panels in identifying who should receive specialist services, because of the 'function' problem of knowing what the services are supposed to achieve. Without clarity of functions, the nature of structures that should enable functions is also at risk. For example, lack of clarity about function led to the increased diversion of one school-based unit into general duties in the mainstream school. This loss of resource to the unit seemed a risky strategy, particularly in the critical early years of the unit's existence. It is therefore important to ask awkward questions about rhetoric that leads to policy without working out the practical implications for the wider system it affects. There is an unacceptable lack of detail in the propositions of some who have the luxury of a moral high ground that is remote from the practicalities of delivering services. This is especially regrettable when, for 30 years (from Kugel and Wolfensberger, 1969 to Wolfensberger, 1995), the principle of normalisation (now called 'social role valorisation') has been a powerful force for change in health and social services. This principle is concerned with recognising human diversity as normal, and proposes how policy and practice may interrelate to enable people who may be disadvantaged by a narrow perception of 'normal', to lead open, valued and fulfilling lives. It appears to have had little explicit impact in Scottish educational provision for pupils with special needs.

The study also showed a need for more networks of teachers, SLTs and psychologists across council boundaries to develop understanding of communication and of autistic behaviour. Staff can feel isolated and discouraged because of the small number of colleagues in their own administrative areas who have insight into their specialism. Much of their knowledge and skill will come from experiential learning because of the paucity of documentation to help them, particularly at the level of daily practice with pupils. The need for their specialist service has been recognised by parents and by local and central government. It now needs support to attain a strong craft knowledge and theoretical underpinning and one essential source of this is its own grass roots.

Banathy's discussions of his original systems approach tended to give pride of place to the 'system-environment' model, which has an interesting resonance with Wolfensberger's (e.g. 1972) 'model coherency' – being clear about what services are intended to achieve, ensuring that they achieve it, and knowing that this is worth achieving in the first place. Reflection on the issues highlighted in this chapter show why this may indeed be the principal point of focus. The study of the units in the west of Scotland indicated little clarity about the system which existed. The 1996 HMI document had certainly shown concern for an area in which support was necessary, but the document and this study have indicated problems of definition, initially of the disorders themselves and, inevitably, of the services set up to respond to them. Perhaps the 'system' aspect of the special services does not really exist yet, other than at the level of the individual school or unit.

There were problems also concerning definition of the environment in which the services were supposed to operate. In recent years, the three state education systems of the UK have been preoccupied with implementing their individual variants on national curricula. It can be argued that one set of curriculum prescriptives for all pupils is not a defensible proposition (Bryce, 1993; MacKay, 1993; MacKay and McLarty, 1999). None the less, this is a characteristic of the 'environment' in which the 'system' of support systems for an ill-defined group of pupils has to operate. It is also an environment in which current assumptions about the nature of support are generic, with little willingness to accommodate other propositions about the nature of service. The system is not clear, and neither is the environment. It is against this backdrop that teachers and SLTs must try to work out policies and practices for collaboration.

Chapter 5
A Collaborative Approach to Extended Learning Support in a Primary School Setting

MARGO MACKAY and MARGARET YOUNG

Introduction

This chapter will outline the principle of collaboration whereby children who have language and other communication difficulties are given access to a number of flexible education settings, where their individual needs may be met in a mainstream primary school. The ways in which the SLT and teachers plan intervention, their roles in delivering an adapted curriculum, and the measurement and assessment of results will be reported, together with a detailed child-based example.

The School

The school is situated in central Scotland and serves a clearly defined area of a town of about 80 000 inhabitants. It was built in 1926 as a secondary school with a primary department. In 1972, following the transfer of the secondary pupils to a new school, the primary department was expanded and is now housed in two buildings on one campus. The school is non-denominational and children come from a wide range of home environments. There is an active parent–staff association and school board.

There are about 350 children, plus 40 children on part-time nursery placements. About one-fifth of the children attend the school on placing requests from parents. In this system of open enrolment parents have the right of choice of school for their child. There are 10 children with records of needs who have complex learning difficulties mainly in the area of language and communication.

The school has 13 classes providing for children aged between 5 and 12 years. There is also an extended learning support (ELS) facility catering for the needs of those children with records of needs.

Principles of ELS

It is now 11 years since the LEA recognised the need to provide a unique education facility for children with complex learning difficulties. The children's main areas of impaired development are those of language, motor skills, organisation and attention control. It was acknowledged that these children are not suited to a traditional special school with a population that has global moderate learning difficulties; neither do they thrive in mainstream schools with standard learning support as they require a more individualised plan of work and access to individual and small group teaching; and so the concept of ELS was born. As we shall see, ELS seeks to provide access to a full curriculum with the resultant benefits of integration.

The ELS facility is a local education authority facility. Each child's placement is supported by a record of needs. The facility can cater for up to 10 children and, although it has been recognised that it is much more beneficial for a child to enter ELS in the first primary class (Primary 1) aged 5, in practice ELS has also met the needs of children who have entered at a later stage. Such late entry tends to follow the failure of a previous placement and/or a failure to identify a complex learning difficulty at an earlier stage.

ELS is designed to provide extensive and specialist provision to children with language and communication disorders in a mainstream setting in order to ensure appropriate and positive integration. The basic elements of the ELS structure are as follows:

Elements of ELS

- Each child is on the roll of the primary school and is fully integrated into a mainstream class.
- The provision of an ELS teacher (ELST) to support children and their class teachers (CT).
- An additional 0.2 full-time equivalent (FTE) teacher to provide cover for the ELST for planning and liaison with mainstream colleagues. In exceptional cases, by negotiating a review of the record of needs, this can be increased as required to meet the needs of specific children.
- The provision of a base room in the school for individual teaching and group work.
- The provision of an SLT as an integral member of the team (0.3 FTE).
- The availability of three support for learning assistants (SLAs) to assist all ELS children educationally and socially, with specific pastoral concern for identified children.
- A team approach involving the children, HT, ELST, the SLT, CTs, SLAs, educational psychologists, parents and other professionals as appropriate.

ELS provides a unique framework for each child according to his or her needs. It provides flexibility in meeting each child's requirements through support in class by SLAs, individual teaching/therapy time, group teaching/therapy with peers both in the ELS base and in class and inclusion in class activities. It provides a secure environment, allowing the child opportunities for planned and informal play as well as a more structured learning environment.

An individual timetable is structured for each child to take account of individual, small group and class settings. Each child is thus provided with a predictable and consistent plan for each day. An example for James, the child we will discuss in detail, appears in Figure 5.1 on page 92.

Developing Collaborative Practice in ELS

For the SLT working in the ELS facility the constraint of working part-time (0.3 FTE) has meant that effective and efficient collaboration is paramount. The SLT and ELST have worked together to provide the following framework:

The collaborative framework in ELS

- Joint development by SLT and ELS teachers of a pro forma for planning the listening and talking sections of the 5–14 curriculum [see Individual Education Plan (IEP), below]. This allows a single language assessment and programme to be used for joint planning of goals and integrated record keeping. Although in principle this is working well, it requires further refinement and expansion to other curricular aspects of learning, e.g. personal and social development.
- Joint planning and running of language groups with follow-up sessions in the ELS facility and in the classroom.
- Inclusion of SLAs in SLT sessions to encourage effective follow-up and feedback.
- Joint meetings with parents to report on progress, evaluate the previous plan, discuss continuing needs and plan the next steps. Parents are also invited to attend individual SLT sessions, in school, if appropriate.
- Regular team meetings to evaluate progress and formulate future plans for the children
- Weekly liaison between ELST and SLT and regular liaison with each child's CT.
- Daily liaison between ELST, CTs and SLAs.
- An annual informal review of each child s record of needs with the whole team.
- Staff development and training for mainstream staff.

Creating an IEP

An IEP is prepared for each child. An IEP is a proactive plan which assists the team in the forward planning for, and the effective monitoring of, children with specific needs. In general, the following steps take place:

Steps in creating an IEP

Collecting background information:
- Data are compiled following regular discussion with the child, parents, CT, SLT, SLAs and other professionals.
- Information is gathered from previous records and reports.

Assessment procedures:
- Observation of child's learning style and social skills in a variety of settings.
- Self-assessment checklists.
- Formal and informal language assessments: norm-referenced, criterion-referenced and diagnostic.

Facilitative approaches to learning:
- Suggested teaching strategies.
- General practical arrangements.

Curricular targets:
- Specific aims for each area of the curriculum.
- Long- and short-term goals.
- Clearly stated methodology.
- Precise resources to be allocated.
- Support required.

Pupil profile:
- Positive features of learning and personal/social development.
- Specific difficulties with learning and personal/social development.
- Learning and personal/social development needs.
- Trends.

The development of the child's IEP is a continuous process involving the child and all team members in a cycle of planning, implementing, reviewing and evaluating. Time scales are set for the achievement of targets, and responsibilities of team members are agreed. The ELST acts as a coordinator in collating data and liaising with team members.

A Child-based Example Using an IEP

In order to demonstrate the use of this procedure we shall consider the example of an individual child called James.

Background information

James was referred for an SLT assessment by the health visitor in June 1991, when he was 3 years old. He was recognised as having severe difficulties in acquiring and understanding language. He received SLT at home, in nursery and in clinic. He also attended a pre-school group for children with special needs. He was assessed by an educational

Time	9.00 am	10.30 am	*(INTERVAL)*	10.45 am	12.15 pm	*(LUNCH)*	1.20 pm	2.20 pm *(INTERVAL)*	2.30 pm	3.30 pm
Monday	SLA support in class	SLA support in class	I N	Hymn practice SLA support	SLT (individual)	L U	ELS base (group)	I N	SLA support in class	
Tuesday	SLA support in class 9.30	ELST and SLT (group) SLA support	T E	ELST support (group)		N C	Swimming SLA support	T E	ELST support (individual)	
Wednesday	SLA support in class		R V	SLA support in class		H	ELS base (group)	R V	SLA support in class	
Thursday	SLA support in class 9.30	ELS base (group)	A L	SLA support (assembly)	support in class		ELST support (group)	A L	Music SLA support	
Friday	ELST support (class)			SLA support in class			SLA support for changing only PE		SLA support ELS base with mainstream peer group	

SLA support in class is not always directed at James, thus affording him the opportunity for independent learning

SLT and ELST may also work with CT in mainstream class

SLA support also required for break times

SLA, CT and James may also call upon the support of ELST at other times

Figure 5.1: Sample timetable for James

psychologist and a child psychiatrist, and the process of compiling a record of his special education needs was begun.

It was difficult to isolate his language/communication problems from his overall cognitive development as he was easily distracted, fluctuating between showing only fleeting attention, to becoming fixed on an activity of his choice. At school age it was recommended that he attend a school for children with moderate learning difficulties. He entered a class of six pupils with complex learning difficulties, most of whom had challenging behaviour. Although it had been recommended that ways of linking him into mainstream education should be actively explored, in practice integration was of limited success and often curtailed because of James's challenging behaviour. James pursued a limited curriculum, but was recognised as having visual strengths and was gradually acquiring literacy skills. He enjoyed extracurricular activities such as swimming, library trips and outings.

The closure of this facility by the education authority meant that James was transferred to ELS at short notice. He entered the ELS facility aged 8 years, 6 months and it was intended that he be integrated into a mainstream class. In practice, this had to be a gradual process as he showed behaviour that was very disruptive in this setting. Initially, James spent much of his time in the ELS base working individually or in a very small group.

James's mainstream class

James is now integrated into a mainstream class of 28 boys and girls of mixed ability. Some achieve high standards of work whereas others require support for their learning and behaviour difficulties. The CT works collaboratively to provide a differentiated programme of work for the children using a variety of teaching methods and groupings. The CT is supported by an SLA for much of the time to enable the children with the greatest level of difficulty to access as broad a curriculum as possible and to help foster positive behaviour.

Assessment procedure

Observation

This is an important stage in the process as it is the means by which information is obtained on how James is learning and interacting in naturalistic settings. Observation checklists are completed by the ELST, CT, SLT and SLAs while monitoring James in three separate settings: in his mainstream class, in a small group and in the playground. Observation checklists for James in these settings appear in Figures 5.2, 5.3 and 5.4 (pages 94-6). Additional observations may be carried out during school assembly and during practical sessions, for example physical education or art and craft lessons. All observations are repeated on a regular basis to ensure accurate and up-to-date information.

Name:	James
Activity/Lesson:	Completing work programme with SLA support
Location:	Mainstream class
Time/Duration:	30 minutes **Date:** June 1997

Personal/Social Skills

Asking Questions —
Asked peer what she was doing with a pencil case. Asked no questions of SLA.

Responses to Questions —
Answered some direct questions well, but did not always respond to questions — became angry when question was repeated.

Eye Contact —
None evident.

Participation —
Reluctant to engage in the activity.

Interaction with Teachers —
Tried to engage teacher's attention by lifting chair, making noises. Responded 'All right' when asked to stop.

Interaction with Peers —
Tended to be negative.

Interaction with SLA —
Worked well for very short periods. Reluctant to answer questions.

Learning Skills

Concentration —
Repeated teacher's instructions; wandered around room, hit himself on head with pencil, shouting 'Ow!' — no attention given so stopped. Drummed pencil; sang to himself — getting louder; talked to himself; swung on chair.

Application to Task —
Completed worksheet. Stood up as soon as SLA moved away — watched adults — jumped back into chair.

Coping Skills —
No difficulty with tasks.

Task Organisation —
Moved from task to task without completing each.

Time Management —
Wasted a lot of time.

Resource Management —
Could not find spelling book. SLA helped him to look. DM did not help — stood waving to other pupils.

Information Seeking —
None
Information Giving —
Gave good information to SLA on activity — spoke in a silly voice.

Attending to Instruction —
Listened only to one-to-one instruction. Did not take completed work to SLA as directed but put it in his tray. He took it out later to give to teacher at an inappropriate time.

Figure 5.2: Mainstream classroom observation

Name:	James
Activity/Lesson:	Speech and Language, Social Use of Language Group
Location:	Tutorial room
Time/Duration:	40 minutes **Date:** June 1997

Personal/Social Skills

Asking Questions —
Lacking ability — not managing to repair when comprehension breaks down.

Responses to Questions —
Often requiring specific directing. Answered therapist's questions appropriately.

Eye Contact —
Very little eye contact with SLT when giving directions.

Participation —
Good participation — keen to volunteer for activities. Initiating ideas.

Interaction with Teachers/SLT —
Responsive although needing prompting to stay on task.

Interaction with Peers —
Agitated with peer — became too physical — looks up to other peers.

Interaction with SLA —
Good relationship with SLA, following well in mirroring activity.

Learning Skills

Concentration —
Variable, short and fleeting, tends to become overexcited.

Application to Task —
Looking for peer approval, wants to 'play to the crowd'.

Coping Skills —
Tends to become restless and fidgeting when unsure.

Task Organisation —
Variable, looked for peer support i.e. waited for peer to take lead.

Time Management —
Not applicable.

Resource Management —
Not applicable.

Information Seeking —
Will initiate with others but tends to be based on fantasy e. g. Superman; 'Have you seen Luke Skywalker?'.

Information Giving —
Very reluctant to talk about self and feelings on his first day at ELS.

Attending to Instruction —
In a small group setting he can attend to instructions — interesting to note that complex language and especially inference is not understood. He never asks for a repetition.

Figure 5.3: Small group observation

Name: James	**Occasion:** 4
Time: Lunch break	**Date:** April 1997

1   Who is the child with?   On his own   √

                                                         With others (age and sex)
         He wandered around on his own at first. He then gravitated to a boy in his
         mainstream class who was also on his own.

2   Did the child initiate contact with others?   Yes   √

                                                                                   No

3   Did the child make physical contact?   Yes   √
         He jumped to grab boy around the neck.   No

4   What is the child's role?

         Leader   Equal Participant   Follower   √
         He followed suggestions of other boy and copied some of his actions.

5   Did the child appear happy/comfortable?   Yes   √

                                                                                   No

6   How do other children react when around this child?

         Reject   √   Ignore   √   Tolerate   √   Engage happily

7   Do others initiate contact with child?
         Rarely.

8   Any other comments.
         He appears to want to join in games of football with class peers but is often
         rejected and so tends to play with the other 'isolated' children.

Figure 5.4: Playground observation

Self-assessment checklists

A variety of pro forma are used throughout the year. These provide a valuable insight into James's changing perceptions of his own strengths and difficulties, reflecting his self-image. An example is included in Figure 5.5.

Discussion of the information gathered

It is in the area of personal and social development that James experiences the greatest problems. The educational psychologist stated that James has longstanding difficulty in making and maintaining peer-group relationships. To a significant extent this may be linked to his

My Name: James   **Date:** February 1998

	Almost always	Sometimes	Never
1. I work hard		√	
2. People trust me		√	
3. I am happy	√		
4. Other children like me	√		
5. I have good ideas	√		
6. My teacher likes me		√	
7. I am well behaved in school		√	
8. I like to say things in class			√
9. I wish I were someone else			√
10. I get on well with other people		√	
11. People miss me when I am not at school		√	
12. I help other people	√		
13. I do not do well in school		√	
14. I like myself	√		
15. I get into a lot of trouble		√	

Figure 5.5: James's Self-assessment checklist

communication difficulties. Although he appeared from an early age to be relatively comfortable in the presence of other children, there seems to have been little interaction with them. He is able to manage some relationships although he does tend to be drawn to more disruptive pupils or younger children. He can be kind and caring to the little ones. He is more comfortable in the company of boys than girls and can be somewhat chauvinistic, describing many activities or objects as 'soppy'. He tends to become angry with friends who do not share his interests or activities. He likes physical play but finds it difficult to allow others to enter his personal space. In contrast, he does not respect the space of others. His imaginative play consists mainly of comic characters or computer-game characters. He tends to direct others in this sphere of play and becomes very frustrated if they refuse to cooperate.

When the play activity is of his choosing, he can display a good level of concentration; indeed he can become absorbed in the activity and difficult to move on. Frequently, James demonstrates fixed, self-imposed routines in his play, for example choosing the same computer game over and over again and playing it exactly the same way each time. This inflexibility is highlighted in his interpretation of rules which he perceives as rigid. Instructions are understood literally with no flexibility. For example, he was told that homework would be given on three specific nights each week, and angrily refused to comply with any deviation to this routine.

Because of his lack of understanding of the pragmatics of language, James often seems rude. He does not tend to modify his speech or his attitude according to his audience. He treats peers and adults alike showing little audience awareness, although he can be well mannered as if to suggest that he is aware of a particular social grace but not always able to access it. He generally accepts adult authority, particularly that of teaching staff, but does not always give the same respect to learning assistants.

In a one-to-one situation James is usually cooperative and works well. He finds it much more difficult in a group situation and tends to be noisy, making inappropriate interruptions and displaying behaviours designed to draw attention to himself. He finds it difficult to attend and listen during group work. In his mainstream class, James tends to opt out of whole-class activities unless he has individual support. At times he appears to attend to and understand instructions or verbal information but at other times he appears unable to listen to or act on information given to him. He does not stay on task and displays many and varied delaying and displacement actions, for example tapping, making noises, making faces or wandering around the room. He can be very disruptive in this situation. At first, James found it extremely difficult to take part in whole-school gatherings but this is gradually improving. Many of James's peers find his behaviour (when he is inappropriately making noises, jumping about and clapping) amusing. James enjoys their attention and reaction to his behaviour.

In the playground, James requires supervision at all times. He moves quickly, tending to climb on walls and railings. He can be difficult to keep in sight. He enjoys playing football but when a game is not being played he tends to wander around aimlessly on his own or becomes physical with other boys. He finds it difficult to wait in line at the end of break.

James's self-esteem, as shown by his self-esteem checklists – see Figure 5.5 – has been increasing steadily throughout his inclusion in a supported mainstream setting. His evaluation of his own strengths and difficulties is generally accurate when assessing his own learning but he tends to overestimate his social skills and seems to be relatively unaware of his own and others' needs in this area.

Formal language assessments

Language and communication assessments are made by the SLT. Assessments used include the Clinical Evaluation of Language Fundamentals (CELF-R UK, Wiig/NHCSS, 1994), the Criterion Referenced Inventory of Language (CRIL, Wiig, 1994), the Word-Finding Vocabulary Test (WFT, Renfrew, 1995), and the Phonological Assessment Battery (PhAB, Fredrickson et al., 1997). Figure 5.6 summarises James's assessment results. This information is gathered over many weeks in order to compile an accurate profile of strengths and development needs and is reassessed annually to record progress.

Test	Age	Results and comments
CELF-R UK	8;6	Receptive Language Score 70 Expressive Language Score 62 Total Language Score 64
CELF-R UK	9;11	Receptive Language Score 83 Expressive Language Score 76 Total Language Score 77
CRIL Pragmatics	8;7	Performance across all pragmatic probes indicates instruction required in all areas. Particular problems with referent and correct pronoun selection.
WFT Renfrew	9;0	33/50 correct. Responses tend to be egocentric, e.g. target 'watering can': response: 'Well I don't know much about these garden things. I don't spend much time in the garden'. Good access of accurate semantic information but not specific words.
PhAB	9;6	All subtest scores within normal limits except for the fluency test (rhyme).

Figure 5.6: Language and communication assessments by the SLT

Education assessments are made by the ELST. James's assessments in the areas of reading and spelling are summarised in Figure 5.7 on page 101.

Categorising Assessment Information Under Curricular Headings

Information is thus collected from a variety of sources and in a variety of forms. The next step in constructing an IEP is to consider and categorise this information under curricular headings. In the Scottish 5–14 curriculum the language strands are listening, talking, reading and writing. Personal and social development are also important. The relevant language points for James are listed on page 100. These help to develop facilitative approaches to learning and the curriculum adaptations and targets necessary for an individual child.

Discussion of Assessment Information

Listening

- Listening is heavily dependent on James's level of attention at different times and on his interest in the task — performance is therefore inconsistent.
- He can understand simple instructions and directions.
- He struggles to process information when it is given in purely auditory form, especially if trying to follow a sequence of instructions or if they involve inference.
- James's semantic system is impaired and he has great difficulty categorising, and forming associations between, words.
- His performance improves with visual support for his memory.

Talking

- James has word-finding difficulties.
- He has problems constructing and sequencing sentences to form a narrative.
- He has difficulties linked to pragmatic language use and therefore often misunderstands what is relevant and the purpose of interaction.
- He may take little regard of his listener's point of view and prefer to communicate on his own terms. He can easily become engrossed in his favourite topics of computer games and comic characters.
- He struggles to adapt to non-verbal rules, e.g. his eye contact is poor, he can be insensitive as to whose turn it is to speak, and he uses inappropriate non-verbal messages (i.e. claps, turns away, gesticulates) about who he is referring to.
- His verbal interaction strategies are poor, e.g. he may use the wrong pronoun, thus confusing the listener about who he is referring.
- He does not give the listener sufficient information, assuming a shared level of knowledge.
- His use of language is rigid, literal and lacking in subtlety. He is egocentric and can be resistant to engaging in language activities that he does not perceive as interesting or relevant to him.

Reading

He reads with expression and demonstrates an expanding sight vocabulary. Although his comprehension is limited to a literal understanding of the text, his word-attack skills are developing well. He is able to find information from a reference text with support. He enjoys reading familiar stories and comic books but shows little awareness of genre. His reading ability is sufficiently developed to allow him to access the mainstream curriculum and is therefore not a focus for intervention.

Writing

He is able to write brief reports and imaginative stories but is more reluctant to write about personal experiences. His handwriting can be rather large and untidy but he is now trying to write more concisely and is learning to link his letters. He is able to write a sentence using a simple word book and can spell some three- and four-letter words phonetically.

Test	Age	Results and comments
Neale Analysis of Reading Ability	8;5	Rate: 8 years Accuracy: 6;5 Comprehension: 6;1
Burt Word Reading Test	8;5	6;4
Vernon Spelling Test	8;5	6;5
Quest Diagnostic Reading Profile	8;5	James demonstrates strong visual skills but poor auditory memory, commenting 'I can't play this game'. He has good word attack skills and an adequate sight vocabulary but tends to reverse familiar words.

Test	Age	Results and comments
Neale Analysis of Reading Ability	9;9	Rate: 8;5 Accuracy: 7;1 Comprehension: 6;9
Burt Word Reading Test	9;9	7;10
Vernon Spelling Test	9;9	7;1
National Tests	9;9	Reading Level A Writing Level A

Figure 5.7: Educational assessments by the ELST

Facilitative approaches to learning

During the assessment procedures, particular note is taken of both the external factors influencing James's education and social achievements and his unique response to his learning and play environment. James's learning style is examined and general practical arrangements, teaching strategies and classroom management strategies are agreed by the team. An example of classroom management strategies is provided below:

Classroom management strategies for James

- Keeping classroom routines as consistent, structured and predictable as possible, with the SLA explaining any essential changes in advance.
- Ensuring resources are clearly labelled and ordered.
- Positioning James in class to minimise distractions and facilitate his focus on the CT or other sources of information, such as the television.
- Prefixing instructions with James's name.
- Using visual prompts such as pictures, personal timetables and charts.
- Giving James extra time to respond to instructions and encouraging any requests for clarification that he may make.
- Being aware of James's tendency to interpret class rules literally and giving him detailed explanations or allowing for a degree of flexibility in the application of rules, where possible.
- Breaking up tasks into small steps with regular feedback and redirection.

Curricular Targets

The next step is to make curricular adaptations and set curricular targets. This section of the IEP sets out the attainment targets for James's language and personal and social development aspects of the curriculum. Methodologies are chosen, resources are allocated to tasks, assessment procedures and criteria are agreed, responsibilities are negotiated and time scales set for evaluation and next steps planning. We have identified a list of resources that have proved particularly useful, and these are listed in an appendix at the end of the chapter.

Personal and social development

As part of James's personal development targets, the following strategies were devised and implemented to facilitate positive social integration for James in his mainstream class:

Personal and social development strategies for James

- Allow James to choose classmates to come to ELS for planned play activities on Friday afternoons.
- Include classmates in a language group in ELS to act as role models.
- Encouragement to join in appropriate group activities in class.
- Encourage a buddy system whereby some of James's peers are specifically appointed to support him in certain tasks.
- Investigate child self-esteem and child interactions in the class
- Structure a peer-group network to create an intensive and individually tailored community around James's needs to give him a safer subgroup in which to acquire and practise academic, social and group skills.
- Introduce circle time by the ELST, the SLT and the CT to enable James to become a valued and accepted member of the class by providing opportunities for the children to develop an appropriately positive regard for themselves and for others and their needs.
- Provide opportunities through circle time for the children to develop skills in cooperation, conflict resolution and social inclusion.

These strategies have been very successful for James and he is beginning to be accepted by his mainstream peer group, which facilitates his inclusion into his mainstream class.

Language targets

Worked examples of the listening and talking targets over three consecutive terms are presented in Figures 5.8–5.10 (pages 104-15).

Ongoing assessment and evaluation provides evidence of outcomes and attainment of targets. This leads to our new aims for the next term. Outcomes are measured using a variety of techniques listed under assessment procedures; i.e. observation in both natural and planned settings, self-assessment checklists and formal and informal language assessments. One of the chief benefits of working in a collaborative team is that often, when the ELS teacher is leading an activity, the SLT can observe, and vice versa. Observation may be documented by checklists or by audio- or video-taping. Pupils are encouraged to assess their own performance in relation to agreed targets.

Pupil Profile

These procedures constitute the IEP, and provide a set of working documents that structure and guide James's education and development. However, there is also a need to summarise the information for those who are not so closely involved with James, such as visiting specialists, and so a summary pupil profile is prepared which provides an overview of the key features of the IEP. This highlights James's most salient development needs and strengths and gives an indication of trends in his progress. Figure 5.11 (page 116) gives an example. These summaries are regularly updated, and are typically reviewed at the start of a school year.

As James's example shows, the construction, implementation, evaluation and development of an IEP is a cyclic process, which maintains focus on a child's changing needs.

Achieving Aims Through Collaborative Practice

Our experience working in ELS has demonstrated to us that time spent in planning, implementing, assessing and evaluating collaboratively is worthwhile and good practice. It can be tempting, when under pressure of time, to 'go it alone'. This, however, leads to a fragmented education experience for the child. By contrast, collaboration brings a cohesive and focused child centred approach that uses the skills and personalities of each member of the team. Targeting learning strands using a variety of methodologies and resources and in different settings promotes the transfer of skills from one situation to another. This ultimately benefits the child's learning experience.

Figure 5.12 (page 117-8) illustrates how the various team members (including parents) collaborate to help James. In a sense, this is one of the most important illustrations in this chapter.

STRANDS FOR LISTENING   Name: James   Date: April – June 1997

LISTENING/ATTENDING	Level I G C	Attainment targets	Learning activity and resources	Assessment evidence for evaluation	Outcome
• Individually • In small groups • In classroom	G A	To sustain attention during 3-minute group discussion	Social Use of Language Group	Observation by SLA	1 (2.6.97)
• To respond to text • To identify the type of text	G	Introduce 'mirroring' technique	In pairs with SLA or peer. Progress from hands and arms to whole body	16.6.97 Good focus, responding well, excellent at following leader	2
	C	To observe in class ability to follow classroom instructions	Checklist	Observed by ELST and SLA	1

PHONOLOGICAL AWARENESS

- To discriminate single sounds words
- Segmentation skills syllables
  + – sounds blending
- Identification of sounds
  initial
  final
  medial vowel
- Identification of rhyme

Note :

James attained Level A in reading May 1997

Spelling 2 years behind CA

*Check phonological awareness

contd.

COMPREHENSION	Level	Attainment targets	Learning activity and resources	Assessment evidence for evaluation	Outcome

• Auditory sequential memory
• Semantics
  <u>concepts</u>
  <u>vocabulary</u>
	I
	G
	C
		To improve broad-based semantic organisation skills by strengthening, building and expanding current system	Memory skills worksheet:
			categorisation
			same/different
			odd-one-out
			LDA cards
			CLIP worksheets (semantics)
			semantic links
				27.5.97 - CELF-R subtests:
				
				1 Word Classes
				  Standard Score (6)
				2 Semantic Relationships
				  Standard Score (7)
				
				Semantic Sorting Assessment
				April 1997 7/15
				June 1997 12/15
				* Check word finding
					3

• Understanding language forms grammatical structures sentences sequence • Ability to comprehend oral information discussion question	A	Target Fruit/ vegetables Clothes Transport Sport Occupations			

Key

<u>Outcomes:</u> 1 = Objective achieved; 2 = Skill emerging; 3 = Objective requires further input; 4 = No noticeable progression.
<u>Settings:</u> I = Individual; G = Group; C = Classroom.

Figure 5.8 i: James's Individual Education Plan (Listening and Talking) April – June 1997

STRANDS FOR TALKING   Name: James   Date: April – June 1997

EXPRESSION	Level I G C	Attainment targets	Learning activity and resources	Assessment evidence for evaluation	Outcome

• Intelligibility of speech
• Semantics
  concepts
  vocabulary
	G
	
	A
		To improve awareness of appropriate/inappropriate volume in speech	Social Use of Language Group
			
			(Week 4) Role Play Situation
				James still using inappropriate volume especially in class — he tends to be too loud	

• Sentence construction
  grammatical structure
  sequence
• Appropriate delivery
  rate / intonation / volume
			— at home
			  — in class
			  — in cinema
			  — at football game
			
			Peer feedback and discussion
				Some increased awareness	3

INTERACTION					

• Turn-taking skills
• Body awareness
  eye contact
  facial expression
  gesture
• Self awareness
	G
	
	A
		To improve turn-taking skills
		
		To improve listener awareness especially with peers
			Social Use of Language Group
			
			— CLIP worksheets (pragmatics)
				Observation
				
				James remains egocentric — tries to distract others to preferred picture. Rarely asks questions. Does not
					2
					
					3

contd.

INTERACTION	Level	Attainment targets	Learning activity and resources	Assessment evidence for evaluation	Outcome
• Audience awareness	I G C			like to admit to having difficulty. Little awareness of how to enter discussion although keen to participate.	
individual					
group		To improve topic maintenance	— video discussion and feedback		4
• Use of language to:	C				
direct		To improve use of appropriate questions	— role play		4
question	A		— SLA/SLT provide good/bad models to discuss	Checklists completed by SLA, SLT, ELST (June 1997)	3
give personal comment		To improve self-monitoring skills	— self-evaluation sheets		3
convey information					
negotiate		To encourage participation in discussion (whole class)			

Key

Outcomes: 1 = Objective achieved; 2 = Skill emerging; 3 = Objective requires further input; 4 = No noticeable progression.

Settings: I = Individual; G = Group; C = Classroom.

Figure 5.8 ii: James's Individual Education Plan (Listening and Talking) April – June 1997

STRANDS FOR LISTENING   Name: James   Date: September – December 1997

LISTENING/ATTENDING	Level	I G C	Attainment targets	Learning activity and resources	Assessment evidence for evaluation	Outcome
• Individually • In small groups • In classroom • To respond to text	A	G	To sustain focus of attention during 6-minute group discussion	Sharp-eye Group Visit by bird watcher	Observed by SLA — much improved — interested in theme	1
• To identify the type of text		C	To improve ability to respond to teacher's instructions	Teacher to prefix instructions with name SLA direct/prompt	Response <u>very variable depending on topic</u>	2
PHONOLOGICAL AWARENESS						

• To discriminate single sounds
  words
• Segmentation skills
  syllables
  + − sounds
  blending
• Identification of sounds
  initial
  final
  medial vowel
• Identification of rhyme
		I	To assess phonological awareness skills	PhAB	All subtest scores are within normal limits except for the fluency test (Rhyme) subtest	1

contd.

COMPREHENSION	Level	I G C	Attainment targets	Learning activity and resources	Assessment evidence for evaluation	Outcome
• Auditory sequential memory	G	G	3 x weeks. To improve semantic knowledge relating to 'Birds' theme.	Sharp-eye Group	Good response to teaching specific vocabulary — excellent recall	1
• Semantics — concepts vocabulary	A	C		Clackmannan bird project		
• Understanding language forms grammatical structures sentences sequence			Improve categorisation and classification	Visit to University for bird watching	Lots of input required on sorting, classifying and categorisation	3
• Ability to comprehend oral information discussion question			Improve ability to identify key information	Semantic links worksheets Bird books from the library — choose favourite bird and identify key information	Progress noted	3

Key

Outcomes: 1 = Objective achieved; 2 = Skill emerging; 3 = Objective requires further input; 4 = No noticeable progression.

Settings: I = Individual; G = Group; C = Classroom.

Figure 5.9 i: James's Individual Education Plan (Listening and Talking) September – December 1997

STRANDS FOR TALKING   Name: James   Date: April – June 1997

EXPRESSION	Level		Attainment targets	Learning activity and resources	Assessment evidence for evaluation	Outcome
		I				
		G				
		C				
• Intelligibility of speech		I	To formally asses word-finding skills	Renfrew Word-finding Test	Renfrew WFT — 33/50 Lots of egocentric responses	1
• <u>Semantics</u> <u>concepts</u> <u>vocabulary</u>	A	I/G	To improve word-finding skills	Reinforce all vocabulary relating to 'Birds' theme as for Listening strand	Requires prompting when completing semantic links	3
• Sentence construction grammatical structure <u>sequence</u>		I	To improve ability to 'write' news	Semantic links worksheets	Thinking rigid	
• Appropriate delivery rate / intonation / volume				Introduce mind maps		2

contd.

INTERACTION

			Setting	Sharp-eye Group	Observation	Outcome
• Turn-taking skills						
• Body awareness						
	eye contact	To improve eye contact when listening to adults/peers		'Birds' topic	Much more aware of the 'rules' and will self-correct	2
	facial expression					
	gesture	To improve regard for others' opinions therefore to be less egocentric	A	'Talk about' worksheets and discussion	Listening to others is improving and is generally more relevant. Some progress noted with eye contact	3
• Self awareness		To improve self awareness and develop a more realistic view of self		— listening — eye contact — relevance — topic maintenance — starting/ending conversations	James is more accepting of self and own profile of strengths and weaknesses	2
• Audience awareness						
	individual	To improve ability to ask and respond to questions				3
	group					
• Use of language to:						
	direct					
	question					
	give personal comment					
	convey information	Self-evaluation sheets			Checklists completed	
	convey information					
	negotiate					

Key

Outcomes: 1 = Objective achieved; 2 = Skill emerging; 3 = Objective requires further input; 4 = No noticeable progression.

Settings: I = Individual; G = Group; C = Classroom.

Figure 5.9 ii: James's Individual Education Plan (Listening and Talking) September – December 1997

STRANDS FOR LISTENING	Level	I G C	Name: James	Date: January – April 1998		
LISTENING/ATTENDING	Level	I G C	Attainment targets	Learning activity and resources	Assessment evidence for evaluation	Outcome
• Individually • In small groups • <u>In classroom</u>	A		To assess visual, auditory and kinaesthetic channels and profile strengths and weaknesses for CT	Coin, coffee bean, stick test	Visual strengths, kinaesthetic OK, auditory weakness	1
• To respond to text • To identify the type of text			To improve listening in class to teacher and peers	Circle time — SLA monitor	Progressing — requires less clarification	2
PHONOLOGICAL AWARENESS						

• To discriminate
  single sounds
  words
• Segmentation skills
  syllables
  + – sounds
  blending
• Identification of sounds
  initial
  final
  medial vowel
• Identification of rhyme						

contd.

COMPREHENSION	Level	I G C	Attainment targets	Learning activity and resources	Assessment evidence for evaluation	Outcome

• Auditory sequential memory
 • Semantics
   concepts
   vocabulary
			To improve ability to listen to information and use in discussions	Circle time
				
				 'Finding-our' game
					Becoming more independent — will volunteer information	

• Understanding language forms
   grammatical structures
   sentences
   sequence
				Paired activities
				
				 Yes/No game
					Looks to CT or SLA for support when comprehension breaks down	2

• Ability to comprehend oral
   information
   discussion
   question						

Key

Outcomes: 1 = Objective achieved; 2 = Skill emerging; 3 = Objective requires further input; 4 = No noticeable progression.

Settings: I = Individual; G = Group; C = Classroom.

Figure 5.10 i: James's Individual Education Plan (Listening and Talking) January – April 1998

Name: James Date: January – April 1998

STRANDS FOR TALKING	Level	I G C	Attainment targets	Learning activity and resources	Assessment evidence for evaluation	Outcome
EXPRESSION						
• Intelligibility of speech			To improve ability to construct sentences and sequence ideas when 'writing' or	Expand use of mind maps for personal and functional writing: i.e. project work	Enjoys creating mind maps	
• Semantics concepts vocabulary					Learning to work well with peer	2
• Sentence construction <u>grammatical structure</u> <u>sequence</u>	A	I/G	mind mapping news	(1) middle ages (2) houses (3) games	Mind-maps helping with story sequence — requires more work with sentence construction	
• Appropriate delivery rate / intonation / volume						
INTERACTION						
• Turn-taking skills			To improve use of appropriate eye contact when speaking/listening	<u>Circle time</u>	More aware — James is now able to use eye contact when imitating and sustaining conversation	2
• Body awareness <u>eye contact</u> <u>facial expression</u> gesture	A	G		CLIP worksheets		
• Self awareness			To improve use of appropriate facial expressions		Over-exaggerates facial expressions and body language	3
• Audience awareness individual group						

contd.

INTERACTION	Level I G C	Attainment targets	Learning activity and resources	Assessment evidence for evaluation	Outcome
• Use of language to direct question give personal comment convey information negotiate		To develop a positive attitude towards girls		Requires more input	4
		To improve use of language for commenting and expressing approval/ disapproval		Will comment — less inappropriate.	3

Key

Outcomes: 1 = Objective achieved; 2 = Skill emerging; 3 = Objective requires further input; 4 = No noticeable progression.

Settings: I = Individual; G = Group; C = Classroom.

Figure 5.10 ii: James's Individual Education Plan (Listening and Talking) January – April 1998

SUMMARY PUPIL PROFILE	Name: James Date: September 1997
Positive features of learning and personal/social development	• Reading skills give access to a wide curriculum • Caring attitude to younger pupils • Generally cooperative given support in class one-to-one • Responds to praise and encouragement • Participates well in PE activities and team games
Specific difficulties with learning and personal/social development	• Difficulty in listening and attending in interactions with others • Inappropriate interruptions and behaviour in group/class situation • Tends to display avoidance behaviour when presented with work which he perceives as difficult • His strongly developed beliefs of right and wrong tend to be rigid, leading to potential areas of conflict with peers and adults
Learning and personal/social development needs	• Needs to focus on listening and attending to information directed at him • Requires to know the structure of his day/week and notice of impending change be given • Monitoring own behaviour • Good role models to display appropriate behaviour and responses • Given opportunities for discussion/role play to understand, appreciate others' responses and perspectives
Trends	• Showing signs of integrating more comfortably into group/class situation • Finding peer relationships difficult • Tends to be possessive of friendships

Figure 5.11: Summary pupil profile

AIMS	SLT	ELST	CT	HOME
Encouraging writing of weekly news Improving narrative structure: beginning, middle and end	Introduce concept of mind mapping to pupil. Produce initial mind map Scribe news story using mind map	Discussion of mind map with pupil and development of strategy of mind mapping as plan for story writing Development of keyboard skills	Encouraging pupil to use mind mapping as plan for news and story writing. Opportunities to write personally, imaginatively and functionally, e.g. write thank you letter to visiting speaker on bird watching	Parent to write weekend news in home–school diary to facilitate discussion of news with pupil
Developing skills in asking and responding to questions	Teach and practise question words: What? Where? Why? How? Appropriate responses to be taught and practised. Questions related to class topic on birds	Role play interview with bird watcher. Asking and responding to questions on birds	Visiting speaker to talk about bird watching. Pupils encouraged to ask questions Visit to local pond to observe birds. Responding to questions from peers about birds observed	Observation of birds in garden. 'Guess which bird I am looking at'. Use of appropriate question words and responses encouraged
Improve word-finding skills and learning of new vocabulary associated with bird topic	Strengthening of semantic system using mind maps and semantic links	Games to help memorise new vocabulary: snap, lotto, word searches, crosswords, etc.	Labelled diagrams for new vocabulary. Frequent use of new terminology	List of new words pinned on wall
Promote good listening and attending to class instruction	Discussion of 'keys' to good listening. Assessment of pupil's auditory sequencing ability. Setting up of circuit of listening stations	Observation of pupil in class. Barrier games to listen to and respond to instructions. Encouragement to visualise instruction	To ensure pupil is looking at her when she is giving instruction. Saying pupil's name before giving instruction. Limiting number of information carrying words	Observation of child's ability to follow instructions at home

Figure 5.12: Team collaboration

contd.

AIMS	SLT	ELST	CT	HOME
Help pupils have a positive regard for self and others	Encourage use of appropriate eye contact for speaking and listening. Improve commenting skills. Use of facial expressions and body language. Planning and participation in class circle time	Observation of pupil's positive and negative interactions with peers in class and playground. Compilation of sociogram to illustrate class relationships. Planning and participation in class circle time	Pupil self-assessment questionnaire to demonstrate pupils' own self image in class. Pupils asked to indicate their choices of companion. Using information collected to form class groups. Planning and participation in class circle time. Encouragement of supportive atmosphere in class.	Monitoring of pupil's self image. Encouragement of positive comments about self and others. Invitation of friends to play

Figure 5.12: contd.

Conclusion

Effective collaboration is hard but rewarding work. Initially, it was found that the ELS functioned as a separate entity in the school, with the children being on a mainstream class register in name only. At that time children rarely left the comfort zone of their base; various professionals including psychologists and SLTs withdrew children to a separate room for therapy or extra support. Today children are fully integrated into mainstream classes. Many of the mainstream children enjoy and benefit from participating in ELS activities. All of the professionals work closely together and the children are in the unique position of being able to access as much or as little support as is necessary at any given point in time. One child recently left ELS to go to his own mainstream primary school, as for him ELS had become a 'safety net' only.

James, our main example, came from the sheltered environment of a special school and yet went on to exceed the expectations of not only himself and his parents but also the various professionals who worked with him. In his first year he progressed at a remarkable rate, especially in relation to literacy. This gave him a great sense of achievement and he later commented that he had 'gone over the top with his work'. It has been rewarding to observe him respond and adapt to his environment and to see him being accepted in a mainstream context. The writers suggest that such rapid and sustained progress will, generally, only be achieved by adopting a collaborative working approach.

Appendix – Useful Resources

A list of resources and materials that have proved useful in the ELS context, some of which are mentioned in this chapter, are given here.

Circle time

Bliss, T. et al. (1995) *Developing Circle Time*. Bristol: Lame Duck Publishing.

Curry, M. (1997) Providing emotional support through circle time. *Support for Learning*, **12**: 126–9.

Galloway, F. (1989) *Personal and Social Education in the Primary School*. Kidlington: Pergamon Education Publications.

Mosely, J. (1997) *Quality Circle Time in the Primary Classroom*. Cambridge: Learning Development Aids.

Social use of language

Kelly, A. (1996) *Communication Skills – Talk About – A Social Communication Skills Package*. Bicester: Winslow Press.

Rinaldi, W. (1992) *Social Use of Language Programme (SULP)*. Windsor: NFER-Nelson.

Rustin, L., Kuhr, A. (1989) *Social Skills and the Speech Impaired*. London: Taylor and Francis.

Semel, E., Wiig, E. (1991) *Clinical Language Intervention Programme (CLIP) – Semantic Worksheets*. Sidcup: The Psychological Corporation.

Warden, D., Christie, D. (1997) *Teaching Social Behaviour*. London: David Fulton.

Learning style

Buzan, T. (1993) *The Mind Map Book*. London: BBC Publications.

Evans, A. (1987) *Reading and Thinking*. Wolverhampton: Learning Materials.

Mitchell, J. (unpublished) *VAK Test*. Communication and Learning Skills Centre.

Semantics and word finding

Barad, D.S. (1983) *All the Games Kids Like*. Tucson, AZ: Communication Skill Builders.

Bothwick, C. (1993) *Semantic Topics*. Newcastle upon Tyne: STASS Publications.

Color Cards – Everyday Sequences; Verbs; Adjectives; Nouns; What's Wrong? Bicester: Winslow.

Mitchell, J. (unpublished) *Classicards*. Communication and Learning Skills Centre.

Sharp Eye (1992) *My World Teachers' Resources*. Aylesbury: Ginn.

Thomsen, S. (1982) *Stimulus Pictures for Assessment, Remediation and Carryover (SPARC)*. East Moline: Lingui Systems.

What Would You Do? Why–Because; Verbal Absurdities. Cambridge: Learning Development Aids.

Syntax and phonology

Dawson, R. (1994) *Story Maps*. Nottingham: NES Arnold.

Semel, E., Wiig, E. (1991) *Clinical Language Intervention Programme (CLIP) – Syntax Worksheets and Morphology Worksheets*. Sidcup: The Psychological Corporation.

What's My Mime? Cambridge: Learning Development Aids.

Assessment

Armstrong, S., Ainley, M. (1988) *South Tyneside Assessment of Syntactic Structures*. Newcastle upon Tyne: South Tyneside Assessment of Syntactic Structures.

Armstrong, S., Ainley, M. (1988) *South Tyneside Assessment of Phonology*. Newcastle upon Tyne: South Tyneside Assessment of Syntactic Structures.

Dean, E., Howell, J., Hill, A., Waters, D. (1990) *Metaphon Resource Pack*. Windsor: NFER-Nelson.

Dunn, L., Dunn, L., Whetton, C., Burley, J. (1997) *British Picture Vocabulary Scale (BPVS)*. Windsor: NFER-Nelson.

Fredrickson, E., Frith, U., Reason, R. (1997) *Phonological Assessment Battery*. Windsor: NFER-Nelson.

Gathercole, S., Baddely, A. (1996) *The Children's Test of Non-word Repetition*. London: The Psychological Corporation.

Muter, V., Snowling, M.J., Hulme, C. (1998) *Phonological Abilities Test*. London: The Psychological Corporation.

Neale, M.D. (1989) *Neale Analysis of Reading Ability*. Windsor: NFER-Nelson.

Renfrew, C. (1995) *Renfrew Word-finding Vocabulary Test*. Bicester: Winslow Press.

Renfrew, C. (1997) *Bus Story Test*. Bicester: Winslow Press.

Robertson, A. (1983) *Quest: Screening*, Diagnostic and Remediation Kit. Leeds: Arnold-Wheaton.

Vernon, P.E. (1977) *The Graded Word Spelling Test*. London: Hodder & Stoughton.

Wiig, E. and National Hospitals College of Speech Sciences (1994) *Clinical Evaluation of Language Fundamentals (CELF-R UK)*. Sidcup: The Psychological Corporation.

Wiig, E. (1994) *Criterion Referenced Inventory of Language (CRIL)*. Sidcup: The Psychological Corporation.

Chapter 6
Collaboration in Mainstream Settings

ELSPETH McCARTNEY

Introduction

The last two chapters have discussed settings where specialist provision is made for children with language and communication difficulties, in language units in Chapter 4 and in an extended learning support setting in a mainstream primary school in Chapter 5. Such settings are characterised by the fact that they are resourced to cater for children with language and communication difficulties, and children are directed to these settings. Because of this, interest and expertise is built up in individual schools, which can become centres of expertise. These factors help collaborative practice to flourish.

However, in 'regular' mainstream schools and nurseries, children with severe language and communication difficulties are only a small part of any school's population, and it is harder to build up good working relationships and collaborate. Difficulties have been recognised. Reid et al. (1996: 61) found: 'joint planning and joint working to be more prevalent in special education facilities than in mainstream schools'. Wright and Graham (1997) also found that collaboration between teachers and SLTs was most likely to occur in special education settings. In view of these findings, it is appropriate to look specifically at issues pertaining to mainstream schools. Although some of the examples in this book have already illustrated good partnerships developing in such settings, the issues are sufficiently important to be considered separately. The systems models outlined in Chapter 1 will be used again to look at collaborative practice, listing problems and discussing solutions at the levels of functions, structures, process and systems environment. The areas discussed as barriers in Chapter 2 and as patterns of collaboration in Chapter 3 will be revisited and refined in connection with mainstream schools.

Functional Issues

Selecting and prioritising children

In Chapter 2, which considered barriers to collaboration, the issue was raised of the difference between education and health services: education services are allocated to all children whereas health services select children for targeted provision. This difference in fundamental functions remains an issue in mainstream schools when teachers and SLTs want to collaborate, and is confounded by issues around resource allocation.

The reasons for educating children in mainstream schools are based on a philosophy of social inclusion. Thomas (1997) outlines the case for such inclusion in terms of social justice, social value and social rights, arguing that an inclusive system is one in which children have a right to attend their community's school by default, rather than by demonstrating their 'readiness' to transfer to that setting. An inclusive school should involve everyone and ensure that everyone belongs, both for the benefits of the children attending and for the overall ethical benefits to society.

As well as social arguments, there are educational arguments in support of children with language and communication disorders attending mainstream schools. HMI (1996: 36) gives a list, although this was a discussion of language-unit children integrating for part of their time in mainstream settings rather than receiving the bulk of their schooling there.

Some advantages of integration:

- children received models of appropriate behaviour and peer language
- there was less dependence on adults
- progress could be reviewed and monitored in the type of settings to which most children would move
- language unit staff remained in touch with the mainstream curriculum
- mainstream teachers remained aware of the continuum of needs related to pupils with language and communication disorder.

It was most effective when there was:

- commitment from senior staff, other staff and parents
- a clear policy specifying the rationale for integration and how it was to be implemented
- a clear definition of the purposes of integration which were taken account of in IEPs
- sufficient time set aside to allow specialist staff to consult with class teachers and each other.

HMI (1996: 36-7)

Such arguments have led to an acceptance of the need to include more children with special education needs in mainstream schools. Government education policy is clear on this point, devoting a chapter in the green paper 'Excellence for all Children' (DfEE, 1997) to how this aim is to be implemented, and the changes that can be undertaken in mainstream and special schools to facilitate the process.

Health service policies that aim to prioritise children to receive services are not easy to accommodate in this context. Where children are to receive education in the least restrictive environment the question of which children are to receive services considered necessary to help them learn is not particularly meaningful. The idea of a child being a 'clinical case' is similarly unhelpful: one aim of educating children in mainstream schools is to prevent their being stigmatised as special or different in the way that 'caseness' implies. The notion of equal access to mainstream schools with a curriculum differentiated as necessary is almost diametrically opposed to the notion of selecting those deemed 'pathological' for service provision. Education in a mainstream setting is one outcome of adopting the principle that all children have the right to receive appropriate services.

However, SLTs find it difficult to accommodate all children who would benefit from services: there are simply not enough therapists to go round. Services that had about six SLTs per 100 000 population (including all adults and children) were reported by RCSLT (1996): Enderby and Davies (1989) had estimated a need for at least 26 SLTs to serve that population number. Figures based on gross population numbers are not very helpful, as they do not consider the ways in which staff are deployed, but the overall difficulties of providing sufficient SLT services to meet demand from education remain considerable. There has to be some way of deciding among the competing demands of children with language and communication difficulties in mainstream schools which respects the need for equal access to services, based on priority.

The way in which this has been achieved in some SLT services is by devising and publishing prioritisation policies. These detail how children are to be assessed and selected to receive SLT attention. Most such scales consider the child's current ability to communicate and the severity of the problem. Other factors such as the prognosis (the predicted future for the child based on knowledge of similar children) and what the research literature says about the probable benefits of intervention might also be taken into account, and sometimes the amount of concern around the child, itself seen as a bad prognostic sign. The factors that apply to individual children are listed and weighted according to severity, and the sum of the weighted scores provides an index of priority for receipt of service. Some of these factors are not known, or involve a fairly subjective judgement, but properly devised scales can capture some of the realities of clinical decision making. As was noted in Chapter 2, such ways of managing demand are not common nor popular in education, which has a remit to provide services to all children, but are used in SLT services, which do not have resources to meet all demands.

Some scales have been devised to allow prioritisation in specialist settings, when all children have some claim to services but resources do not allow all to have provision. Others, relevant to this chapter, have been devised to include mainstream schools. An influential approach developed in Sandwell, West Midlands, UK, was designed to be used for children with special needs across school settings (Sisson et al., 1994)

Prioritisation scheme

The following questions would be answered:
- does the child have feeding or swallowing difficulties, or use an alternative or augmentative communication system?
  If so, three points are automatically added.

Alternatively,
- how severe is the child's language difficulty?
  Score 0–3

For all children,
- how effective is the child's communication?
  Score 0–3
- what ability has the child to change?
  Score 0 (poor prognosis)–5 (good prognosis)

Total scores give the priority for service, with
  0–2 = low priority
  3–5 = medium priority
  6–11 = high priority

Sisson et al. (1994: 5-6)

Such prioritisation schemes do not get over the basic problems of lack of SLT staff and demands for service outstripping supply. They do, however, make the basis of decision making transparent, and are open to public scrutiny. They protect equality of access to SLT services for children, although this may mean in practice that many children have an equal right never to receive services. At least such open decision-making procedures can be defended or challenged, and are open to public debate about distribution of resources.

It is likely that service prioritisation procedures will take place across a whole SLT service area, and can be applied to a whole education authority area. Since they are based on child need, individual schools will have varying amounts of contact with SLT services over time according to the particular children they have on the roll. This makes it difficult for individual teachers and SLTs to build collaborative partnerships, which require good social relations. Much activity will no doubt remain at the cooperation and coordination levels outlined in Chapter 3. Helpful documents of the kind devised by Honeyfield (1997a), also cited in Chapter 3, will be required to ensure that everyone is aware of what is going on. At all levels, documentation may have to be extensive to try to take the place of face-to-face discussion.

Education provision versus deficit models of practice

At a functional level, most children are not selected for mainstream schools because of language and communication difficulties, or any other kind of difficulty. Teachers in such schools have not elected or trained to work with children who require special help, although most will have received information on special education needs as part of their pre-service training. The mainstream model of practice is usually based on adapting the curriculum to a child's needs rather than identifying and targeting problems within the child, and children with 'labels' attached to their difficulties may make teachers fear that they do not have the specialist knowledge or resources needed to tackle such problems. However, they may have the support of special education needs coordinators (SENCOs) or learning support teachers to provide help and advice.

In Chapter 3 the importance of inservice training was stressed to overcome some of these difficulties. Inservice work can make teachers and SLTs more confident that they understand the relevant contexts, and can be an efficient use of scarce time if group work is used effectively, and SENCO back-up provided. Chapter 3 gave examples of the topics on which inservice courses might focus, although clearly it would be sensible to plan in detail to take account of local needs.

Models of interprofessional collaboration

As discussed in Chapter 2, many staff will have limited experience of working across professions, and perhaps different ideas about how joint working can operate. Some time spent clarifying individuals' knowledge and expectations can be useful. An example from Bothwell (1997), a practitioner on a postgraduate course reflecting on practice, illustrates the point (see page 126).

Bothwell's example suggests that these mainstream teachers had a generally informed picture, but individual responses indicated some misconceptions. Two members of staff thought that an SLT would always give priority to speech difficulties over language difficulties, and two were unsure of an SLT's qualifications. One thought that the SLT was employed by the education authority (possibly confused by the education authority's contribution to supply of SLTs for children with records of special education needs in Scotland). Otherwise the teachers were fairly accurate. A model of shared teaching and collaborative planning was desired, although there had been little formal experience of it. Bothwell was able to use this information, together with additional information from the deputy head, the learning support teacher, the SLT manager and the SLTs who had worked in the school previously, to improve collaborative practice.

Teachers' expectations of SLT in mainstream settings

Bothwell (1997) surveyed staff in an all-age mainstream primary school in a rural area, where she was taking over a post as SLT. The school had 189 primary pupils, three with records of need. The school had had SLT input for some time, mainly on an extract basis with some review meetings, with 14 children on the SLT caseload. Questionnaire responses were obtained from the four teachers who worked with these children, and one each from the deputy principal and learning support teacher, answering questions about SLT services.

Four respondents knew that SLTs required a degree to practice, and all could list at least one subject that would have been studied. Five knew who employed SLTs, but one thought the education authority employed the school SLT. All could name three places where an SLT would work, and give examples of who might refer. All (accurately) noted themselves as possible referral agents.

'True or false' questions elicited a fairly accurate appreciation of children's problems and SLT's priorities – all agreed that children would usually have developed all speech sounds before entering Primary 1 aged about 5 years, and that children of above-average intelligence could have language difficulties. Two, however, felt that speech problems would always take priority in an SLT's caseload.

Staff were knowledgeable about reasons for referral to SLT services, all mentioning speech problems, and three also mentioning language delay, one communication problems and one social problems. They gave a wide variety of helpful examples of information that an SLT might like to have before seeing a child for the first time, but only three mentioned information on education performance. All suggested that teachers would be among the people implementing language programmes devised for children. Five teachers felt it was important that teachers should have training on working with children with communication problems – one said this was of some importance, three very important and one essential.

Two had had some inservice training; two had had some training in their degree programmes, and the other two had had no training beyond watching an SLT work. Five wanted further training, and one did not reply. The training suggested included two respondents who wanted to watch an SLT at work, one who wanted information on lip and tongue positions, one who wanted knowledge about language delays and disorders and how to teach speech sounds, and two who wanted information on how to help particular children. One wanted an inservice day, and two wanted joint planning and consultation time.

Bothwell (1997: 15-17)

Social barriers

When SLTs are present in schools only as occasional visitors it can be hard to build the kind of social relationships that are important for joint working, and that help to develop the mutual trust and respect seen as a hallmark of good collaborative practice. This in itself will probably be a limiting factor in developing collaborative work. DiMeo et al. (1998) make this point. Their working definition of collaborative practice involves: 'a high level interpersonal working relationship, similar in many ways to a personal friendship' (p. 50). In the same way that it is not possible to become personal friends with all colleagues DiMeo et al. consider it unrealistic to expect that all professionals will become true collaborators. Interpersonal dynamics will be relevant, but in many mainstream situations an important issue is simply lack of shared time to develop partnerships. DiMeo et al. (1998) argue that interpersonal 'comfort' is an essential aspect of such good working relationships, and that this takes time both to develop and maintain. If this time is not available in mainstream settings, good and indeed professional working relationships can still develop, and a civil and courteous approach can pertain. However, it is not reasonable to expect a high level of collaboration to develop, and many relationships will remain at the level of compliance and cooperation. Even using the robust definition presented in Chapter 2 (p. 33) collaboration may not be achieved. Egalitarian relationships and mutually determined goals may be developed, but SLTs and teachers will have difficulty in coming together to implement them.

These interpersonal and dynamic aspect of collaboration are important, and may be underrepresented in many policy statements. They probably require more consideration than is usually given in organisational contexts, and are important in maintaining staff morale and continued levels of commitment. The provision of time and continuity to sustain good social interactions should play a large part in the planning of service organisation and service delivery. Mainstream schools without such time may be prevented from developing good collaborative practice. They will have to fall back on good documentation, and shared record keeping at classroom level will assume a large place in ensuring good joint working relationships.

Structural Issues

Timing and location of service delivery

The need for SLTs to collaborate by working in mainstream schools rather than extracting children from them has been stressed, and is easy to justify on educational grounds. However, the logistics of providing such a service can be difficult, and are particularly daunting in mainstream schools. Because such schools tend to be relatively large they have to be tightly timetabled and organised. This means that teachers and SLTs can find it hard to find opportunities to meet and discuss children, and headteachers can find it difficult to facilitate this process. The demands of the curriculum can be heavy, and it can be problematic to find time to plan a differentiated curriculum for an individual child while meeting the needs of the other children in the class. The difficulties discussed by Taylor (1997) in Chapter 3 illustrate this problem, and her partial solution describes what is probably a typical compromise.

However, the overwhelming problem for SLT services is not finding liaison time with teachers in the mainstream school, but simply of getting to the schools at all. The example of prioritisation difficulty presented in Chapter 2 occurred, as stated, when two additional full-time SLT posts were funded to provide a service to 105 children across 40 schools; and when the therapy service as a whole had requests to provide service to children in more than 70 schools, some with only one or two children requiring SLT input (Luscombe and Shaw, 1996). It is difficult to see how such large numbers of locations could be serviced with such small staff numbers. The difficulties are severe and widespread. In the RCSLT's response to the green paper 'Excellence for all Children' (DfEE, 1997) it supported the principles of inclusive education but highlighted the costs to SLT services that increasing inclusion will bring. The college notes:

> Where children are focused within one special school, SLTs can concentrate their resources both in terms of contact with the individual children and in terms of teaching staff so that the provision of appropriate communication environments becomes more feasible. To spread the same children throughout geographically distant mainstream schools places considerable strains on the resources and organisation of SLT services (RCSLT, 1998: 8).

The examples given by the RCSLT (1998) are of problems in organising safe eating and swallowing procedures for children with severe physical difficulties, and in providing the knowledge to support technical communication aids – both areas where SLTs have particular expertise to offer. However, the difficulty of providing any kind of service, let alone a collaborative service, with resources spread too thinly across a large number of schools clearly applies to many children with language and communication problems.

This is in no way an argument against inclusion, but a practical point about resources. The relatively poor collaboration found in mainstream schools is probably a result of overstretched staffing, rather than a difficulty about mainstream settings per se. It is difficult to run a thorough-going, inclusive approach to children's language and educational needs, or to share expertise across a variety of settings, when both SLT and teaching services are so thinly stretched. Careful time planning at a local level of the type advocated in Chapter 3 is clearly necessary, but limits will remain unless more SLT input can be found.

Management structures

The need to effect good collaboration in mainstream settings once again raises the issue of management structures, and the need for managerial planning between health and education services at all levels was stressed in Chapter 3. At the level of the school, the school-based service-level agreement was outlined as a useful tool for planning many aspects of collaborative working. However, if large numbers of mainstream schools are involved, it is hard to see how it would be practical to organise a school-based service-level agreement for each. It is more likely that a general template would be needed, based on a formula agreed at NHS trust and education authority level, which gave an equitable distribution of SLT resources across children and spelled out what would be available. The level of SLT service would be based on children's needs, and so would vary considerably over time in any one school. However, such an education authority-based service-level agreement together with prioritisation measures as exemplified above would give individual schools and SLT services a reasonable picture of the amount of SLT time available, the roles and functions to be carried out and which expectations were to be met. The planning level would thus move up from the individual school to education authority level, although implementation and monitoring of the service-level agreement would still take place on a school-by-school basis.

An alternative approach has been outlined by Lennox and Watkins (1998) which focuses on opportunities for collaboration. These authors were part of a team that developed a model aimed at collaborative working which would meet the communication needs of children and involve school staff, SLTs and parents. Language support teachers and SLTs used both their overlapping and distinct specialist skills to develop a service. The model of service delivery involved inservice education; and also joint planning, implementation and evaluation of group work in schools where children worked on language goals. These language groups were designed to help schools concerned with the early stages of meeting children's identified needs. The whole programme is interesting, but a significant structural issue emerges in that the project set up criteria which schools had to meet to enter the scheme.

These are clearly reasonable criteria, but only seven schools met them. As well as the small number of SLT staff available, which restricted the size of the scheme, there were similar limits on school staff – resource problems do not just affect SLT services. These constraints put considerable pressure on individual teachers and therapists, and funding issues continued to limit development of the scheme.

Entry criteria for collaborative service delivery

Schools had to:
- identify language as a priority on their school development plan
- want to develop their special education needs policy with particular reference to speech and language
- identify a number of pupils with speech and language needs who would benefit from group work
- designate a teacher to take responsibility for running groups two mornings a week
- have adequate accommodation for small group work.

Lennox and Watkins (1998: 13)

This approach offers a realistic appraisal of the local situation, and can help highlight the realities of practice. It also presents managers with choices (rather hard choices) about where to put scarce services, and alerts decision makers to some of the difficulties caused by resources not following exhortations to collaborate. The limited number of children offered a good service did benefit, and this is no doubt more effective than offering an inadequate service to a large number. The obvious step forward – that all children should be offered an adequate service – will, however, depend on additional resources.

One response to limited facilities developed in education contexts is the notion of clusters of services, usually schools, collaborating to share scarce resources to meet special needs. Gains and Smith (1994) give examples of various possible models. Some of these incorporate specialist services (their examples are learning support teachers) supporting schools in a variety of ways.

Models of school clusters

Gains and Smith (1994) list seven possible models of how clusters of schools could use specialist staff:

- pooling of school staff, for example for staff development purposes
- information exchanges via inter-school working groups
- skills exchanges via the direct 'swapping' of school staff (an uncommon model)
- direct funding of specialist help by a cluster of schools
- 'carousels', where specialists rotate among schools
- 'magnets', where children travel to specialised bases, such as IT bases
- 'caravans', where the specialist or specialist equipment is transported around schools.

Gains and Smith (1994: 96)

Most of these models could be extended to include SLT services, which currently rely mainly on 'carousel' approaches. The interesting structural aspect is the need for managerial cooperation across school boundaries to form some core organising group. If such clusters of schools are being developed, there is a need to coordinate school organisations with NHS trust organisations in order to incorporate SLT provision effectively into ongoing local developments. The possibility of schools accessing SLT services through technology such as video conferencing is becoming more realistic (Charter, 1997).

Curriculum structures

As discussed in Chapters 2 and 3, the implementation of national curricula has caused some tensions between SLT and education services, but the resulting focus on communication in the classroom has been productive. SLTs have adapted and fitted their language aims to curriculum structures. This has allowed joint planning and record keeping, and has facilitated collaborative work.

However, there are still questions to be asked about the limits of SLTs' collaboration in curriculum issues. SLTs have expertise in all aspects of communication difficulty, which can extend to aspects of literacy. Many children with reading and writing problems have well-attested difficulties in aspects of language, particularly those pertaining to phonological processing (Torgesen et al., 1994), and some children with speech and language difficulties are at risk of reading failure (Stackhouse and Wells, 1997: 16). SLTs have been involved in developing and implementing education programmes to develop children's skills in phonological processing (Gillon and Dodd, 1997).

Because of this expertise, there is a rising demand for SLT input to be extended into the area of early literacy development and the prevention of reading failure (Gorrie et al., 1998), which could mean SLTs working with children who had no overt language or communication difficulties. At present, as Gorrie and colleagues comment, hard-pressed SLT services may be avoiding, or at best restricting, SLT involvement in the development of reading, for fear of being overwhelmed by a deluge of referrals. Consultancy approaches and inservice work are going on, with SLT involvement in the construction of training packages for teachers and programmes for children. Beyond this, there are unresolved issues about the types of children who should be referred (only children with language and communication difficulties in addition to reading difficulty? Children who had such problems in the past but whose problems had resolved?). Once again, decisions might best be considered at a functional level to help clarify the issues posed by the literacy curriculum as a structure. Decisions need to be made at an NHS trust and education authority level, with clear prioritisation measures in place, to ensure equality of provision and availability of expertise.

Process Issues

Opening a statement or record of needs

As Chapter 1 outlined, there is currently a difference in the ultimate funding responsibility for SLT provision for children who have statements or records of special education needs compared with those who do not. SLTs' disquiet with this situation was also noted. There is also unexplained local variation in the number of children with statements or records of need, as mentioned in Chapter 2 in relation to Scottish specialist provision (HMI, 1996: 14) and as noted in England and Wales for all types of children (DfEE, 1997: 38).

The direct relationship between SLT funding and the possession of a statement or record of needs is unfortunate. The overall thrust of education policy, as discussed in Chapter 1, is to recognise that the vast majority of children with special educational needs will have these needs catered for in mainstream schools without a full record or statement being opened. An individual child's special needs are also seen as reversible, with requirements for additional support reducing as the child becomes more able to engage with the curriculum. This is particularly appropriate for children with language and communication difficulties, whose problems frequently change over time. Their problems can reduce, or less happily commute into literacy or emotional and behavioural difficulties as the child matures (Davidson and Howlin, 1997). Children who do not require or who no longer require a full record or statement should be able to access services as well as those with the process complete. It would be a great pity if funding arrangements fail to recognise this, and if receipt of SLT services depends on the possession of a statement or record. This would go against the grain of current education and social policy. Resolution of this area as promised in government policy statements (see Chapter 1) is required.

Planning for SEN

Discussion of barriers to collaboration in Chapter 2 predicted that fewest problems would occur at a process level where consideration is given to children's individual interactions with a service as they enter, access provision, and leave. The use of IEPs gives a focus to joint planning, and teachers and SLTs are both comfortable with the ideas of specific adaptations and work plans for individual children. There is no particular difficulty pertaining to mainstream education, and curriculum differentiation approaches are appropriate.

There is still a need to share information on action that can help children. Materials prepared jointly by teachers and SLTs at a practical workshop session are published in Anderson et al. (1990). They were designed for children aged 3–7 years in mainstream schools, and cover speaking, listening and building confidence in communication. Activities and planning examples for older children are contained in Merritt and Culatta (1998). Programmes of work are not discussed in this book, but there is a need to further develop and share useful curriculum-based programmes and techniques.

Systems-environment Issues

Parents have received special consideration throughout this book, and once again mainstream schools seem to be an area where particular care is needed so that parents' needs can be understood and their contribution welcomed. As with the other issues in relation to mainstream schools, resources and opportunities to include parents are limited, and SLT services have expressed concern at the lack of routine access to parents when working in mainstream schools compared with special settings and health clinics (Reid et al., 1996: 77). Policy initiatives to include parents in mainstream schools have tended to be concerned with structural issues such as ensuring parental input to boards of governors, rather than concentrating on functions or increasing informal staff–parent contact. However, mainstream schools are often well integrated into their communities, and parents may find them more convenient to access than special units – the access problems outlined by the parents interviewed by McCaughey (1997b) in Chapter 3 may not arise. The potential for including parents in education planning is great.

The suggestions about including parents in collaboration are fairly obvious and common sense. Parents' meetings and home–school diaries feature in many settings, and SLTs can contribute to these as well as teachers. A school- or education authority-based service-level agreement with an SLT service can write in the amount of work of this kind expected. Apart from the few schools that have a specific home–school teacher attached, schools almost exclusively ask parents to visit the school rather than teachers visiting the home. This may again be a result of practical aspects of resources and timetables rather than because of policy issues. SLTs have more flexible timetables, and often undertake visits to children's homes to talk to families. It should be possible for collaborating professions to make good use of such opportunities, making sure that information is exchanged among the collaborating team and parents, and that parents know that this will be the case. There are also opportunities for SLTs to see parents outside of school terms in clinic settings, and these can be capitalised on. Clarifying funding for such services may require some managerial time, but the resulting benefits to families and children are potentially great.

Conclusion

The particular difficulties for teachers and SLTs collaborating in mainstream settings have been traced through all four levels of the systems model, and are seen to be great. There are some differences in philosophy between health and education which particularly impinge on mainstream settings, and there is a real need for supra-school decision making to set patterns for work across many schools in an education authority. However, most of the difficulty for teachers and SLTs collaborating in mainstream settings does not arise from differences in philosophy or models of good practice. Difficulties are largely a result of resource limitations. It is perceived as very expensive for SLT services to supply services to children in mainstream schools, because of the scatter of such children and the limited number of staff employed: it is seen as very expensive for mainstream teachers to have sufficient time made available to collaborate with visiting SLTs, because of the needs of other children in their classes.

Lacey and Ranson (1994: 80) recognise this, stating:

> Where there is a commitment to an holistic view of pupils with SEN, the effort involved in getting a team to work is repaid with time saved, resources expanded and with quality of the service enhanced. This is not, however, achieved without considerable effort. Professionals need to understand each other's roles, experience and expertise. Time must be given to know the extent of the role of a [specialist ... and] to know about the strengths and weaknesses of the person filling that role. Only when this understanding is achieved will resources be used well so that pupils receive a unified response to their needs. There is no suggestion that specialisms are unnecessary but the greatest benefit for the child is derived only when the relevant skills, knowledge and understanding are shared. There is no short cut.

Unfortunately, it appears that resource limits have tended to mean that SLTs and teachers in mainstream schools have been asked to short-cut the collaboration process. Enough is known about the process of collaboration to realise that it flourishes where there is sufficient liaison time given to understand one another's context. Services have made heroic efforts to manage tiny resources, employing prioritisation schemes, documentation, inservice work and group work to good effect. But there are restrictions as to how much further individual services can spread resources. If mainstream education is to be the usual form of education for children with language and communication difficulties, as education and social policies suggest, and if many children in mainstream education have language and communication difficulties, problems will not be solved by stretching resources ever thinner. A solution to the SLT funding problem, as promised in current legislation, is needed, and probably also an increase in resources. Collaboration in mainstream schools may then approach the levels achieved in special services.

Chapter 7
Stammering Children in Schools

ROBERTA M. LEES

Introduction

This chapter will look at the child who stammers in the classroom, as the stammering child often needs a different approach from children with other types of language and communication difficulty. First of all, the term 'stammering' needs to be defined. The terms 'stammering' and 'stuttering' are synonymous, with the former term being used more often by British authors whereas American and Australian authors are more likely to use the latter. 'Stammering' will be used here to refer to a 'disorder in which the "rhythm" or fluency of speech is impaired by interruptions or blockages' (Bloodstein, 1995: 1).

These interruptions may take the form of repetitions of sounds, sylla-bles or short words or prolongations of a sound, e.g. 'Whe-e-e-e-e-n can I go?' Blockages occur when the flow of air or voice is stopped and the speaker is unable to produce the desired sound. If this occurs at the beginning of an utterance the speaker would seem to have a delay before initiating speech. The disorder can and usually does vary in severity from day to day and sometimes over a very short period of time, depending on circumstances: for example, a child may speak fluently to another child in class then may stammer when answering the class teacher's question. The reactions of the speaker to the perceived inter-ruptions in speech play a considerable part in determining the extent to which the speaker is handicapped by this condition. Some individuals who stammer will react by changing the words of the sentence to avoid a word on which they thought they would stammer, e.g. 'My favourite fruit is an (apple) – pear', or by pretending not to know the answer to a question. Some stammering adults are so skilled at changing words in the sentence that stammering is never heard. In young children this is more unusual as they do not have an adequate range of necessary vocab-ulary to do this effectively. Their best disguise is not to speak at all; thus stammering children may be very quiet in the classroom. Stammering children may also use extraneous movements, for example blinking or foot stamping, in the belief that this helps them to pronounce words. In addition, emotional reactions such as fear and embarrassment about speaking may occur, especially if the child is teased about the problem by other children. The stammering child then needs sensitive handling to prevent a deterioration both in speech and in his or her reactions to talking.

To obtain the optimum results in education, in communication skills and in maintaining a positive self-esteem with stammering children, a team approach to management is needed, with the class teacher and SLT playing integral roles in the team. When the SLT and the classroom teacher first come into contact concerning a stammering child, the perceptions and beliefs of both towards stammering should be examined. The extent to which stereotypical beliefs can affect behaviour is uncertain, but it seems likely that the beliefs held by each will influence any intervention programme for the stammering child. Thus the perceptions that the teacher and the SLT have of the stammering child will influence the amount of success the child experiences in school and beyond school. This chapter will examine teachers' and SLTs' perceptions of stammering children, the reported educational attainment of these children, and recommendations will be given on how teachers and SLTs could work together to the benefit of stammering children. A practical example is presented to illustrate some of these features.

Teachers' Perceptions of Stammering Children

A number of studies have been carried out mainly in the USA into teachers' perceptions of stammering children. The findings are relatively consistent and suggest that teachers tend to stereotype stammering children as being shy, tense, insecure and quiet. In an early study, Woods and Williams (1976) asked a number of participants, including a group of teachers, to rate four hypothetical individuals (male and female stammering adult; male and female stammering child) on 25 opposite adjectives (for example, 'nervous' versus 'calm') which had been selected from personality traits found in previous studies. There was strong agreement in the group that the stereotypical person who stammers is submissive and non-assertive, being tense, insecure and afraid to talk to people. The study was replicated by Woods (1978), who obtained very similar findings. Using a similar methodology, Horsley and Fitzgibbon (1987) noted that both primary and secondary teachers in Britain rated hypothetical stammering children more negatively than 'typical' children and that the judgements of girls who stammer were more moderate than those of boys. All of these results were relatively independent of the amount of exposure to individuals who stammer. Lass et al. (1992) and Silverman and Marik (1993) found that groups of teachers most frequently ascribed the adjectives 'shy', 'insecure' and 'quiet' to hypothetical stammering children and adults. Similar adjectives were also used by special educators (Ruscello et al., 1994) and by school administrators (Lass et al., 1994) to describe hypothetical individuals who stammer. More than 80% of these respondents knew someone who stammered but had not necessarily received any formal teaching in the disorder. Crowe and Walton (1981) constructed an inventory of teacher attitudes towards stammering and found that teachers with a greater knowledge of stammering showed more desirable attitudes towards stammering. However, the teachers who displayed more favourable attitudes were less likely to have a stammering child in their class at the time of completion of this inventory. So, it would seem that exposure to stammering is not a necessary prerequisite to developing a stereotype about the disorder. White and Collins (1984) suggest that listeners use their own experience of temporary dysfluent speech and its accompanying emotions to infer the personality of the 'typical' stammering person.

Whatever causes these stereotypes to develop, and however they are assessed, there is a generally consistent finding that stammering individuals are viewed as insecure, tense and shy. Admittedly, ways of assessing these attitudes and stereotypes do encourage respondents to generalise, but the consistency of the findings does suggest that teachers are likely to view and to react to stammering children as if they were shy, insecure and anxious. It is difficult to estimate the effects of this on the child's behaviour and performance in school, but it would seem likely that many teachers would excuse stammering children from oral participation in class in order to avoid upsetting them.

This stereotype is particularly unfortunate because the available evidence does not support these perceptions. A vast amount of research has been conducted to investigate the personality of the person who stammers. This work has been conducted on children and adults who stammer and the results do not support the perceptions of the stammering individual as being shy and insecure. Bloodstein (1995) summarises much of the results of this research with the comment that 'there is little conclusive evidence of any specific kind of character structure or broad set of basic personality traits that is typical of stutterers as a group' (p. 236).

SLTS' Perceptions of Stammering Children

The perceptions of the SLT who is working with the stammering child are also important. If clinicians do not enjoy treating the stammering child or feel inadequate in their knowledge of the problem, then they are unlikely to be able to positively encourage collaboration with the classroom teacher to obtain successful outcomes with this client group. To obtain further information on clinicians' attitudes towards, and knowledge of, stammering and its treatment, Cooper (1975) developed the Clinician Attitudes To Stuttering (CATS) inventory, which contains 50 statements to which the clinician responds on a five-point scale ranging from 'strongly agree' to 'strongly disagree'. Using this inventory St Louis and Lass (1981) found that more than 50% of 1902 students of speech and language therapy, both undergraduate and postgraduate, in 33 states of America, agreed with statements that attributed feelings of inferiority, psychological problems and problems with social relationships to those who stammer. They also agreed with the statement that stammering individuals have specific personality traits. Cooper and Cooper (1985), using the CATS inventory to compare the attitudes of SLTs from throughout the USA over a 10-year period, found that the number of respondents who agreed that stammering individuals have psychological problems reduced from 44% in 1973 to 34% in 1983. There was, however, no change in the clinicians' responses to the statement that most stammering individuals possess feelings of inferiority (more than 60%), and in more than 50% of cases in both studies clinicians agreed that there are personality traits characteristic of stammering clients.

Again, no supporting evidence exists for stammering clients having different personality traits. It is possible that the development of these attitudes could be culturally based. Therefore, Cooper and Rustin (1985) compared the attitudes of SLTs in the USA and the UK again using the CATS inventory. In general, they found agreement in attitudes between the two groups, with more than 50% of both the American and British clinicians agreeing with the statement that stammering individuals have a feeling of inferiority and that stammering clients possess characteristic personality traits. One disturbing finding was that both American and British clinicians agreed with the statement that clinicians are not adept at treating stammering. Thus therapists had negative attitudes towards treating this client group and many had viewpoints about the personality of the stammering client despite a lack of empirical evidence to support these.

Using a different approach to the assessment of attitudes, Horsley and Fitzgibbon (1987) included student SLTs in their respondents and found that when asked to rate hypothetical stammering individuals on opposite adjectives, the stereotype did weaken as students progressed through their course, supporting the belief that education can change stereotypes. It is difficult to assess attitudes accurately; but more attempts to elicit attitudes and feelings of confidence and competence of SLTs working with stammering clients would give some indication of the likelihood of success. One way of increasing the knowledge and with this the confidence of SLTs with this client group is to provide more postgraduate education in the disability. When therapists feel confident in their knowledge of this topic they convey this confidence to others, creating a more positive attitude around the stammering child.

Research on Education Attainments of Stammering Children

Stammering children have been found to experience difficulties in schools in studies across several continents and over a period of time (McAllister, 1937; Andrews et al., 1983). In an early study, Williams et al. (1969) carried out two investigations to examine differences in the academic achievement of 12-year-old stammering and non-stammering children and to compare changes in academic achievement level that occurred from age 10 to age 16. Using the Iowa Test of Basic Skills (Lindquist and Hieronymous, 1964), which gives scores on vocabulary, reading, language, work study skills and arithmetic, they found the median score values for the non-stammering children to be higher than those of the stammering children. In language skills there was a 6-month difference between stammering and non-stammering children at age 10, but this had dropped to 1.3 months at age 16, suggesting that the stammering children tend to 'catch up' with their non-stammering peers. On a test of arithmetic skills Schulz (1977) found no significant difference between stammering and non-stammering children in Germany. There have been a number of studies on the reading abilities of stammering children covering a period of more than 60 years. Nippold and Schwarz (1990) reviewed the literature and concluded that 'while it is clear that some stutterers experience difficulty learning to read, the contention that stuttering children, as a group, are more likely to have reading problems than their non-stuttering peers is neither supported nor refuted by the literature' (p. 175). The authors comment that little is known about the effects of various teaching methods on stammering children's reading achievement. Do stammering children have more difficulty, or experience more anxiety, with a phonic approach that encourages them to sound out letters? In one approach, *Jolly Phonics* (Lloyd, 1992), the child is encouraged to repeat the first sound in the word. This would not seem to be an appropriate method for the stammering child who may have difficulty controlling the number of repetitions. Nippold and Schwarz (1990) suggest that approaches which focus more on the enjoyment and utility of reading may be more compatible with the needs of some young stammering children, especially those with additional language problems and anxiety about oral communication. Thus, until further information is available, the issue of the most appropriate method of teaching reading will largely be the choice of the school, although the speech and language therapist may be in a position to discuss some possible modifications of the programme with the teacher. This would be particularly relevant in the case of stammering children with additional language and communication problems. A number of stammering children do have additional problems with speech sound systems (for example, the child says 'tat' instead of 'cat' or 'wed' instead of 'red'). Louko et al. (1990) found that almost 40% of stammering children had such additional difficulties in comparison with 7% of non-stammering children.

The frequency with which stammering children have additional language problems (for example, problems with finding words, grammar or word order) is uncertain. Nippold (1990) summarised the results of research in this area and concluded that:

> Although the evidence is not convincing that stutterers as a group are more likely than non-stutterers to have deficits in these areas, it is clear that some stutterers do have concomitant speech and language problems that may bear some relationship to stuttering (p. 51).

Children will vary in their reactions to these additional problems but these may contribute to reading difficulties or feelings of anxiety when asked to read aloud in class. It is helpful if the reading material for the child is well within the child's linguistic capacity, so that the child is not 'pushed into' stammering because the material is too complex. The SLT is in a position to give the class teacher information on the stammering child's sound system and language abilities so that reading material can be selected with this in mind.

Courses for Teachers

As stammering occurs in only 1% of the population, it is likely that many teachers will never have had a stammering child in their class or will have had very few. It is also likely that some SLTs will have treated comparatively few stammering children as they represent a small proportion of the work of the clinician. However, there are now specialist centres and teams of SLTs specialising in stammering in some parts of the UK as well as in other countries. As SLTs do have considerable information on stammering, it is generally assumed that the SLT will 'tell' the class teacher something about stammering, thereby effectively placing the therapist in the role of the 'expert', as discussed by McCool in Chapter 8. Stewart and Turnbull (1995) include comments from a teacher who reminds us that the SLT's advice to teachers tends to be based on this expert model and is taken from the viewpoint of the child as an individual rather than as a member of a social group. This is a valid criticism as SLTs have often extracted the child from the class and thus have seen the child only as an individual and have not seen how the child reacts in a larger group setting.

It seems logical to assume, however, that giving the class teacher some information about stammering in general may be a useful first step in working collaboratively to help a specific stammering child in a social setting. A number of authors suggest that this type of 'information giving' is best carried out as part of the teacher's pre-service or as an inservice course (Yeakle and Cooper, 1986; Lass et al., 1992; Silverman and Marik, 1993). The kind of information given tends to be 'factual', for example explaining that 1% of the population stammers and that this occurs in a ratio of about 4:1, male: female, and discussing the probable effects of stammering on the individual in terms of social, personal and educational development. The way children react to stammering is also very helpful information, and gives teachers some understanding of why these children behave as they do in the speaking situation. Pindzola (1985) describes signs that can be useful indicators of stammering for teachers, as outlined in the introduction. For example, the child might remain silent in class, giving the impression of being quiet or shy or may substitute words for others, look away while speaking or pretend to think during pauses.

This is useful information for teachers, but courses that include all of this material are time-consuming and one could legitimately question how many busy teachers would have either the time or the inclination to attend such a course, especially when one considers the low prevalence of stammering. Although such courses would not be needed by all, Stewart and Turnbull (1995) have organised half-day groups for teachers, parents and stammering children. The authors recognise that a longer group would probably be more beneficial, but in practical terms they appreciate that they are more likely to have maximum numbers on a shorter course. In this course, as well as the whole group meeting together, there is also a teachers' group, a parents' group, a teachers' and children's group and a parents' and children's group. Everyone receives information on stammering, often using the stammering iceberg analogy (Sheehan, 1975). This considers all of the overt symptoms that one can see (for example, extraneous body movements) and hear (speech dysfluencies) as being 'above the water'; but the child's anxieties and fears about speaking are not so readily observable and are thus 'below the water'. The extent to which the child has anxieties about speaking will be reflected in the level of the 'water line', which will vary from child to child. In addition, everyone in these groups actively participates in discussion, brainstorming sessions and observation 'games'. In this way parents, teachers and children can all work together to gain a better understanding of stammering, look at the problems stammering can cause and discuss practical ideas on how stammering may best be managed. This is very much an experiential and thought-provoking course, which the authors have informally evaluated, and the 'responses from parents and teachers suggested that some felt the knowledge they gained to be the most important factor, for some it was the insight they felt they now had, while others mostly valued the practical ideas' (Stewart and Turnbull, 1995: 142).

This type of approach would certainly encourage a high commitment by parents and teachers, but is it only committed parents and teachers who would attend anyway? It would also seem sensible to discuss listeners' reactions to stammering, including impatience and embarrassment (Dalton and Hardcastle, 1977), and attempts to avoid or limit the conversation (Rosenberg and Curtiss, 1954). It seems likely that more information on the types of reactions often encountered would help teachers to feel that their own reactions are not unusual and would also help them to change their reactions to more helpful ones. Certainly, giving teachers information about the nature of stammering could help to increase their confidence when dealing with this client group.

The British Stammering Association (BSA) in 1996 produced a very helpful video and information booklet, A *Chance to Speak*, to help teachers deal with a stammering child in their class. The video chronicles the problems faced by a child who has just entered secondary school and is required to answer the register and make a speech in class, and who experiences teasing by the other children. The teacher is first of all shown as being unhelpful in her responses to him (for example, hurrying him), then, after she has taken advice, she responds to him in a more helpful way. The video (lasting 12 minutes) can effectively portray to teachers the importance of the teacher's support to the stammering child, and good advice on reacting to the stammering child is given to help the teacher. The accompanying booklet discusses the overt and covert symptoms of stammering and gives more detail about dealing with the stammering child in class and useful attitudes to adopt. The teacher is advised to build up the child's confidence and to encourage the child to take part in all activities, but to provide an 'opt-out' for the child who really cannot cope with speaking in class. There is also some useful information on teasing and bullying, oral exams and career advice. Teacher attitudes are also targeted with teachers being advised to look beyond the stammer and avoid responding to their perceptions of stammering children. This complete package from the BSA would form a good source of information and would encourage informed discussion.

Sharing Information

Although it is useful as a basis for discussion if teachers have some basic information about stammering in general, the main concern of any teacher must be how to deal with a specific stammering child in his or her class. The child should be referred to the SLT, who will assess the child and make detailed notes about the child's background. On the basis of this information, the SLT can decide on a management programme for the child. Some authors (Ryan, 1984; Peters and Guitar, 1991; Manning, 1996) suggest that the SLT gives the teacher an overview of the child's therapy programme and its rationale so that teachers will have a better understanding of how to interact with the child, and will be better able to give information to the SLT on how much the child participates in class. For example, it is helpful to share notes on whether the child offers information, asks questions or only answers questions; when stammering increases and decreases (for example, does the child stammer more or less when reading aloud, or does the child change the words of a reading passage?); the child's progress in school; and the reactions of the child's peer group to him or her. With this sharing of information the SLT can gain a better picture of the child in a social setting, which can be particularly important if the therapist usually sees the child in a one-to-one setting. The teacher then also becomes part of the child's management programme.

Stewart and Turnbull (1995) also suggest that it would be useful for an SLT to visit the child's classroom if this is at all possible to gain some idea of the atmosphere in the class, how much talking is permitted and expected, and to meet the stammering child's friends. Questions may arise, such as: does the teacher view the child as a normal child who happens to stammer, or as a stammering child who must be shy, insecure and have any of the other personality traits that teachers typically ascribe to this population? In relation to this, does the teacher listen to the content of the child's speech or to the dysfluency? It would also be useful for the teacher to visit the base where the child has therapy, and to observe the therapist working with the child, provided the child is agreeable to this. This could also be done when the speech and language therapist visits the school. The teacher would also gain some idea of the atmosphere being generated in the therapeutic situation as well as the aims and objectives of therapy. In some cases it might be surprising to teachers that the aims are not always fluency and that rewarding the child for participation in the class may often be more important than fluent participation. This type of sharing of information is not particularly difficult when the child is in primary school but becomes more problematic when the child is in secondary school with a different teacher for each subject. At this stage the child will probably be able to indicate a teacher with whom he or she would like the therapist to consult. It is particularly important at this stage to build a discussion around the child's personal profile and to discuss the child's participation in oral subjects. Currently, in national English exams candidates are required to give an individual talk and to take part in discussion. One of the criteria used to assess the individual talk is fluency, although it is possible that this could have more than one interpretation. It could be very difficult indeed for the stammering child to achieve this criterion. In assessment of discussion skills, candidates are required to contribute relevant responses and ideas. Again, the stammering child could be disadvantaged if unable to initiate speech quickly enough to produce a timely response to what is being discussed. The stammering child may also lack the pragmatic skills necessary to take an active part in discussion. Hayhow (1995: 31) cites Weiss and Zebrowski (1991), who used a

'Discourse Skills Checklist' (Bedrosian, 1985) to obtain information from classroom teachers. They found that twice as many non-stammering children as stammering children routinely used a number of the discourse features such as 'disagrees with others', or 'able to make requests for repetition or clarification'. If the participation of a stammering child is so limited, it would seem that he or she could be disadvantaged in this form of assessment. Stewart and Turnbull (1995) suggest that the SLT should write to the appropriate examination board to ensure that the child is not penalised, but this still leaves a problem for teachers on how to assess an oral exam with a stammering child. More discussion between the two professional groups would be useful here to reach agreed marking criteria in these circumstances.

Helping the Child in Class

As a result of descriptions of schooldays by stammering adults, much has been learned about helpful reactions of teachers to the stammering child. A number of authors (Van Riper, 1973; Gottwald et al., 1985; Manning, 1996) provide useful advice to teachers who have a stammering child in class. LaBlance et al. (1994) summarise most of this information by saying that the class teacher can help the stammering child in three ways:

- by providing a good speech model
- by improving the child's self-esteem
- by creating a good speech environment.

The advice is usually along the following lines:

Helpful advice for classrooms

- It is often helpful to call on the stammering child early to read, answer questions and so on, to avoid a long period of anticipation during which time he or she becomes increasingly anxious with a possible resultant increase in dysfluency. The child should usually, however, take part in all activities, as failure to do so could create harassment and teasing from his or her peers. If the child gives a long answer to a question, thereby increasing the probability of dysfluency, the content of the answer may become obscured because of the dysfluency. In this case the teacher could usefully paraphrase what the child has just said, thus giving the child's words increased importance (Manning, 1996).
- The teacher should remain calm, avoiding 'unhelpful' body language such as stiffening, losing eye contact, turning away, showing anger and so on (Gottwald et al., 1985). One of the problems here is that when asked to maintain natural eye contact it is all too easy to stare, particularly if the listening teacher is embarrassed or ill at ease.
- Similarly, teachers are advised to speak slightly slower to the stammering child and to slow the conversational pace. For most people this is

extremely difficult and requires much practice to achieve a decrease in speech rate without sounding abnormal. However, it is possible for teachers to slow the conversational pace by leaving a slight pause after the child has finished speaking. If the child is aware of his or her dysfluency, the teacher is also advised to have a discussion privately about stammering with the child and avoid the conspiracy of silence that so often develops, possibly because of the teacher's lack of knowledge about the disorder or attempts to save the child embarrassment. This open discussion between teacher and child can be very helpful and if handled sensitively can make the child feel 'special' and willing to contribute in class with someone whom the child perceives as an understanding teacher. Van Riper (1973) suggests that the teacher allows the child to read along with other children and finds ways of increasing the stammering child's self-esteem.

There is no doubt that the teacher's attitude can do much to aggravate or alleviate the dysfluency of a stammering child. By creating a relaxed, open atmosphere in the classroom where individual differences are not penalised, the teacher can help to give the stammering child confidence to speak and express opinions which in turn can help to prevent a problem becoming a handicap.

Dealing with Teasing and Bullying

There is some overlap between teasing and bullying as both can involve name calling. Generally, however, teasing is viewed as annoying behaviour designed to create a response from the recipient. Obviously, if the recipient likes the teaser, the teasing may be accepted without any negative response. Bullying, while also involving name calling, can also include making fun of someone's disabilities, physical aggression and isolating someone.

Stammering children are vulnerable to teasing and bullying by virtue of the very fact that their communication skills are obviously different. A number of authors offer advice on how to handle this problem. Peters and Guitar (1991) encourage the child to try to disarm the teaser by such comments as 'I know I stammer and I'm going to speech and language therapy for help'. They practise role play with the child so that the child has the opportunity to calmly and openly admit to his or her stammering in a friendly environment before facing the outside world. This type of acceptance does suggest that the child requires a certain degree of maturity. They also involve the teacher by requesting that he or she tells the teaser that such behaviour will not be tolerated. When teasing becomes bullying there is always the danger that the child will be afraid to tell anyone, but if the class teacher or SLT suspects this, action must be taken immediately. Stewart and Turnbull (1995) discuss the use of a publication, *Don't Pick on Me* (Stones, 1993), which was written for children to help them help themselves when being bullied. In this book children are encouraged to assert themselves and develop 'inner power' to help them cope with the bully. Policies on bullying are now generally available in most schools.

Mooney and Smith (1995) investigated the amount and effects of bullying on stammering children. They developed a questionnaire which was sent to adult members of the BSA and obtained a 30% return (n = 324). Their results showed that 82% of these adult respondents reported being bullied at some time in their lives, the age of most prevalent bullying being 11 to 13 years followed by 8 to 10 years. The most common form of bullying was name calling, followed by threats, physical bullying and rumour spreading. A high percentage (93%) reported that the bullying was often related to their stammer. As the authors point out, this is a retrospective study based on the memories of the respondents. Nevertheless it does show how the problem of bullying and the relationship of this to their stammer is perceived by them. If a large number of stammering children are being bullied, it is difficult for them to respond to this verbally; thus other means of managing this problem must be considered.

The BSA in 1995 produced a pack, *Bullying and the Dysfluent Child in Primary School*, the aims of which are 'to create a safe and productive learning environment for children who stammer' (p. 5). Thus the focus of the pack is the classroom climate, not the child who stammers. A series of useful classroom activities, suitable for 7–11-year-old children, is provided. These activities, which can be incorporated into the curriculum, include activities to encourage children to work together, talk to one another, negotiate, confront difficult issues and experience pressure. There are also debriefing sessions when the children give feedback on the activities. The ideas presented for these activities and the ways in which the children provide feedback are imaginative and would appeal to many children, not just those who stammer. The pack also contains strategies based on assertiveness training for dealing with bullying, although further training in assertiveness would be helpful. This pack can be used by the teacher alone or by the teacher and the SLT. Some of the activities do lend themselves to a joint approach.

An Example of a Joint Approach

To illustrate how a joint approach may work in practice, a detailed example dealing with one child is presented:

A joint approach

Peter, aged 8 years and 6 months, was referred to the author by his general practitioner, who commented that his peer group was now noticing his 'speech problem' and was teasing him. In terms of Peter's age this was a late referral as the chances of successful intervention are better the earlier the child is referred after the onset of the stammer. In Peter's case, his mother reported that his stammer started when he was 2 years old. When Peter was first seen he talked in a mature, insightful way about his stammer, describing his lack of concern about it until shortly before his referral, when he was being mimicked and bullied by older children at school. He was able to provide the following, fairly typical information about his stammer. He stammered more when he was required to make a short speech in class, talk to strangers or talk to people who either didn't like him (based on his perception) or who laughed at him. His concept of people not liking him seemed to be based on their non-verbal reactions to him, especially if these suggested discomfort, e.g. looking away when he was speaking. He did comment that he spoke more fluently with his family, when reciting poetry and when feeling confident. What was particularly remarkable in this case was his insight and ability to verbalise his feelings so clearly.

When assessed, Peter was found to stammer on about 10% of words uttered, although typically the severity did vary, with less stammering being heard when reading than when conversing with the SLT. He tended to repeat speech sounds, syllables and words and he also prolonged sounds. However, there was no evidence of his ever having blockages on sounds. Accompanying his stammer he had some extraneous movement of his feet, dilation of the nostrils and eye closure. Peter's speech rate was slightly fast and he had discovered that if he spoke more slowly he could control his speech more easily, although he stressed that he did not wish to speak abnormally slowly.

He was very keen to participate actively in therapy to improve his fluency, and both parents were also anxious to be involved in therapy. His parents were given information about stammering, their questions were answered honestly and the therapeutic aims were discussed with them. These were threefold:

*   increasing his confidence in himself (and in speaking)
*   slightly slowing his speech rate to give him more feeling of 'control'. This involved a slight slowing of his speech rate while maintaining normal rhythm and intonation. This meant, as he said, that his speech did not sound abnormal
*   preventing the development of speech fears, with a possible resultant avoidance of speaking.

To help achieve these aims, the involvement of the class teacher was discussed with Peter who readily agreed to this. Peter's school was a considerable distance from the SLT clinic and therefore it was not practical for the SLT to visit the school, so the first of a series of phone calls was initiated. His class teacher was keen to ask questions about stammering in general and Peter's stammering in particular. She found the variability in severity to be one of the most confusing aspects of his stammer. She was able to supply information on Peter's willingness to contribute in class and to confirm that he did not seem to be avoiding answering questions in class at this time. She had not heard him reading alone as all reading was carried out in groups: a system that was to Peter's advantage. She was asked if she would privately discuss Peter's stammer with him so that he could tell her what for him were the most helpful ways of responding to him when he stammered. The aims of therapy were explained to her and she felt she could help to build Peter's confidence in himself. The teacher was happy to cooperate in the management of Peter's stammer and she was given the clinic telephone number so that contact could be maintained.

Over the next few months Peter showed gradual but not necessarily steady progress. Stammering is so sensitive to outside events that progress is not always linear; for example stammering can and did increase when Peter was on holiday from school, as his routine had been disturbed. Gradually, however, he gained more confidence in himself, especially after taking part in the school play, where he was fluent, and winning the school poetry competition. He was also achieving success on the rugby field: one of his great interests. Simultaneously, he was gaining much more speech control by slowing his speech rate, although his increase in confidence would also contribute greatly to his new-found fluency. Peter's speech in the SLT clinic was very fluent but he remarked that he would like reminding to use his speech control outside. His parents, who accompanied him to therapy, readily agreed to do this for short periods each day and, with Peter's agreement, his class teacher was again contacted. The teacher was asked if she could, for a short time each day, use a 'secret sign' to remind Peter to use his speech control in class. The teacher discussed this with Peter and they decided on the teacher coughing being the 'secret sign'. Peter's good relationship with his class teacher ensured the success of this approach as he was happy to be reminded by her in this way.

Over time and with changes of teacher, phone calls to the school were instituted to discuss stammering with the new teacher, answer any questions on this topic and discuss the aims of therapy. Peter remarked that he was happy to talk openly to his teachers about stammering, allowing him to feel more comfortable in class.

Now, at age 11 years, he is fluent most of the time, confident about speaking and no longer being teased or bullied. He has not developed any fears about speaking and does not avoid speaking situations. In this case, Peter, his parents and his teachers have been given some information on stammering by the SLT and Peter has felt able to talk openly about this problem. This combined approach, with the teacher and the parents feeling confident about their own reactions to Peter's stammer and Peter being actively involved in his own programme, contributed significantly to the successful outcome in this case.

Conclusion

It is worth noting that Lloyd and Ainsworth (1954), while commenting on the necessity of teacher cooperation for successful therapy, stated: 'It is reasonable to assume that the ease with which this co-operation may be secured and the degree to which it may be expected will be related to the knowledge and training of the classroom teachers and to the attitudes they now hold' (p. 244). This comment is still applicable today. With increasing knowledge of this disorder SLTs are in a good position to give or arrange access to useful information for the classroom teacher and for both then to work collaboratively to the advantage of the stammering child.

In addition, Ramig and Bennett (1995) acknowledge that with therapists having increasing case loads and with personnel shortages, it is likely that collaborative/consultative models of intervention will in future be viable alternatives to the traditional 'extract' model. Although these would provide financial reasons for the SLT and class teacher to work together, there are more compelling therapeutic reasons. If SLTs extract the child, they are hoping to effect some change in the child which will generalise to social situations with which the child is faced. By attending to and enlisting the cooperation of others in the child's environment the generalisation of change becomes more likely. Nevertheless the attitudes of both clinician and teacher do need to be positive, as it seems unlikely that the stammering child will experience lasting benefits without the support and understanding of those in his or her environment.

Chapter 8
Collaboration with Parents

SUSAN McCOOL

Introduction

In a book about collaboration in the classroom, what place is there for a chapter concerned with relationships between professionals and parents? This chapter is based on the view that collaborative arrangements in the classroom both have an impact on and are influenced by links extending beyond the classroom into home and community environments. Professionals collaborating among themselves for the benefit of any child have a responsibility to acknowledge and promote a role for parents in the joint activity.

Working with parents is a complex area. The first part of this chapter attempts to unravel some of the issues facing SLTs attempting to work with parents in an education setting. The second part of the chapter looks at issues involving parents in the therapist–educator framework. The rest of this book describes the complexities of collaboration in the dyad of therapist and teacher. Here, the focus is on the additional implications of bringing another player into the relationship.

Despite the complexities, schools are the scene of many innovative efforts to forge ahead with collaboration involving parents. The efforts of one school will be described, with an analysis of how in practice there are always further steps to be taken.

Collaborating with Parents in an Education Setting

The SLT in education is working at the interface of the two different systems of health and education as discussed in Chapter 2. In many matters, daily practice requires a careful balance of two philosophies and negotiation of the expectations of each. In any circumstances, institutional and organisational matters have an important influence on the success of attempts to work with parents (Pugh, 1989; Crais, 1991). Management support is essential, in the form of resources and clear endorsement of the necessary alterations in working practice.

There are two main organisational issues for the SLT collaborating with parents in an education setting:

1   The therapist has to satisfy two different systems that the proposed collaborative action is worthwhile; each of them requiring justification on different aspects. Health employers require the therapist's practice to be outcome-based and prioritised. Collaborating with parents has to be defended in terms of efficacy. On the education side, therapy services are purchased to meet the identified educational needs of pupils. It has to be shown that work with parents is necessary to meet the child's educational needs.

2   The therapist must ensure that activities involved in collaboration with parents are acceptable to the host, that is, education setting. Further, issues may arise when the brand of collaboration promoted by the education setting is not consistent with the therapist's approach. These issues can arise out of the differences in perspective between health and education staff, an area that is discussed below, as a development of the points raised in Chapter 2.

Involving Parents in Collaboration between SLT and Educator

Collaboration between the SLT and parents, although an important focus, is not the whole picture. For the same child, the SLT will have links with education staff; and the parent and educator will form their own relationship. The network is represented in Figure 8.1.

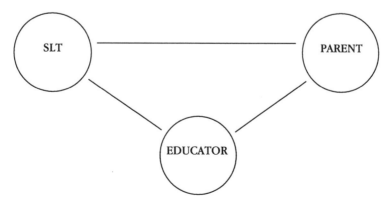

Figure 8.1: Network of separate links between therapist and parent, educator and parent and therapist and educator

Gascoigne (1995) suggests that it is wrongfully simplistic to make the assumption that professionals form one group and parents form another and that one unified collaborative link is easily achieved. Instead, it is argued that the parent is often required to have quite different links with each of the professionals involved with the child. The reality is that the relationships are complex, multiple and variable. There can be differences in procedures and protocols between health and education agencies, arising out of their different philosophical bases. The text that follows examines the different models of working with parents and the divergence that has led to dissimilar orientations and expectations.

General Approaches to Working with Parents

The model proposed by Cunningham and Davis (1985) has had widespread application in both health and education settings. Its definitions are descriptive, based on qualitative analyses of the relative roles assumed by the key people. Each of its components will be described below – the expert, the transplant and the consumer models.

The expert model

In this model, the professional assumes all control over the process of intervention, deciding what information to seek from or give to parents. The parent is not likely to be actively involved in service delivery.

Although this model carries with it the imperative for the professional to deliver well, it is clear that the intervention is unable to benefit from the valuable information about the child's circumstances that the parent could have provided. Similarly, the parent's understanding of the process will be limited and possibly distorted.

The transplant model

In this approach, the professional acknowledges a role for parents in the intervention process. Under the guidance of the professional, the parent carries out some activity with the child.

There is a degree of risk in this model that excessive demands may be placed on some families if the professional does not take account of their resources and capacity for involvement. This is particularly likely in disability services where a range of professionals may each have their expectations. Additionally, closer involvement in intervention programmes also brings to parents more responsibility for the outcomes of the venture. Not all parents will be ready to bear that responsibility with the perspective of professional detachment.

The consumer model

In this model the parent is viewed as an informed consumer of the services offered by professionals. Parents are in control of the decision making, and the role of the professional is to listen to parents and advise on the options available. It is suggested that the advantages of this approach are that the parent is likely to feel in control, less dependent, more informed and ultimately more satisfied with services (Hornby, 1995).

Although the consumer model was intended by its original proponents to most closely approximate the ideal of partnership with parents (Cunningham and Davis, 1985), its interpretation and uptake have led to criticism and caution. Hornby (1995) warns that, taken to the extreme, it can lead to professionals abdicating their responsibilities by allowing parents to make choices without the appropriate guidance and information. A further criticism is that in public services, and especially in special needs provision, scarcity of resources renders parental choice making largely untenable (Sayer, 1989). Further, some detractors comment that the emphasis on individual choice engenders competition and possibly conflict between the users of a service, thereby reducing the power they might have had to change events if they had worked collectively (Sallis, 1988).

The models of working with parents that have been described offer a useful framework for all professionals who wish to reflect on their approaches. However, the concept of involving parents continues to evolve. It is in that development that a divergence emerges between therapy and education services. Models that are influential in each sphere are described below.

The SLT Perspective on Working with Parents

SLTs are trained to work with clients of all ages, whose services are provided in a wide range of settings. The need to work in a spectrum of contexts spanning education, health, social work and voluntary provision generates among therapists an appreciation of multi-agency relationships. There are influences from many disciplines, principal among which are psychological, medical and social models.

Psychological models

SLTs are strongly influenced by the theory of applied psychology and counselling. Their understanding of parents' reactions may be based on the continuum model of coping with grief proposed by Kubler-Ross (1969). In that model, the initial reactions are of shock and denial, and from there various stages lead towards acceptance. It is now felt that parents may re-experience earlier stages at particular points in the child's life. More recent models have stressed parental adaptation (Gargiulo, 1985; Bicknell, 1988) and ways to consider the coping strategies parents employ (McConachie, 1994).

Therapists are often closely involved in the lives of families long before a child starts school, and the mutual expectation of ongoing close links may become firmly established at that time. Those expectations may persist despite changing from one therapist to another or one service setting to another.

Medical models

Most SLTs are employed by health agencies, and as a result their training and practices are influenced by the medical model of intervention. In that model, the child is regarded as having an impairment, which becomes the focus of attention. A diagnosis is made after assessment, with the resulting identification of specialised services to address the impairment.

There has been some criticism of the application of the medical model to the lives of children with impairments (Beazley and Moore, 1995). It is said to ignore the imperative on society to minimise the effects of the impairment, by instead locating the problem solely within the child. Yet, some practitioners consider that it offers a clarity of focus that leads towards well-defined measures of outcome, hence ensuring quality services.

In recent years, health services have adopted a focus on preventive health and public education. In this context, it becomes legitimate for health professionals to include in their remit activities to promote the support and wellbeing of their clients' families and carers. In that sense, work that is part-influenced by the medical model can begin to address the social approaches outlined below.

Social models

The social network model

The social network model will be familiar to therapists' social work colleagues. It is founded on the idea that work with any client in any setting should incorporate an understanding of the client's world from the client's point of view (Seed, 1990). Applied to families, this model leads to an acknowledgement that environmental forces will have a higher impact on the child's development than will the influence of professionals. The practitioner's role becomes facilitative, aiming to promote existing strengths in the social network and facilitating the family's adaptation to events (Appleton and Minchom, 1990).

The theory behind social network models can be traced to three separate models of family functioning (Hornby, 1994), each of which offers some insights that are useful for professionals to reflect on.

The transactional model

The transactional model is derived from the work of Bell (1968) and Mink and Nihira (1987). The child's development is believed to occur in a context of ongoing interplay between a changing individual and a changing environment. Therefore, the family will be influenced by the child as well as having an influence on the child. It follows that the nature of the child's impairment will determine how the family members are affected and the characteristics of the family members will have an effect on the child's functioning and development.

The ecological model

The ecological model (Bronfenbrenner, 1979) is a complex model. Briefly, it proposes that the social environment's influence on families with a disabled member is on several levels, including the extended family, the services available and community attitudes and resources. The suggestion is that each level needs to be considered to fully understand the family context.

The family systems conceptual framework

The family systems conceptual framework was developed specifically to aid understanding of family influences for children with disabilities (Turnbull and Turnbull, 1986). The framework consists of four interdependent areas: family interaction (intra- and extra-family), family resources, family functions and family lifestyle. From a family systems perspective, the goals of any intervention are to identify the family's needs and resources, find the services and support required for meeting those needs, and help families access those means (Dunst et al., 1988).

Several models have been cited as influential in encouraging professionals to include a social perspective in their approach to families. Overall, services are called to recognise the child within a family that is in turn within its own community context. Particularly at the pre-school stage, speech and language therapists have been working increasingly closely with families, using approaches such as the Hanen Early Language Parent Programme (Girolametto et al., 1986, 1993). In the Hanen approach parents are recognised as being the child's primary language facilitators. Parents are led in a series of group workshops and home visits that incorporate video-taped interactions between the parent and child. Parents, therefore, are adopting much more active roles in their children's communication development from an early stage. It seems likely that their expectation of close involvement will persist into the school years.

Having reviewed the psychological, medical and social models that have had an impact on therapists' perspectives, the next section looks at education.

The Education Perspective on Working with Parents

In Chapter 2 of this volume McCartney highlights the differences between education and therapy services. The influence of those differences has also extended into the area of working with parents. Schools are organisations that allocate resources to meet identified special needs. Collaboration with parents in education has evolved in a way that addresses those practical requirements. Some commentators suggest that work with parents has tended to be focused on the exigencies of practice rather than guided by theory or policy (Atkin and Bastiani, 1988). In fact, some consider that this is rightly so (Wolfendale, 1983). Typical in the literature are descriptions of roles parents might fulfil. For example, Morgan (1993) lists eight roles: recipients of information, governors, helpers, fundraisers, experts, clients, co-educators and, finally, consultants. There are various models that attempt to provide defining frameworks in education (e.g. Lombana, 1983; Kroth, 1985; Bastiani, 1989; Wolfendale, 1992). Those models also have firm grounding in practice, looking at possible activities and roles of parents and teachers. The most recent model claims to be a synthesis of the previous work (Hornby, 1995).

Hornby's (1995) model is a diagrammatic representation of the various needs of parents and teachers balanced against their possible contributions to joint practices (see Figure 8.2). The possible roles and needs of parents are arranged in hierarchies according to the proportions of parents likely to be involved. The model also incorporates a dimension charting the amounts of time and expertise required by either party in the various endeavours. It is Hornby's recommendation that his framework is used by each school to generate a checklist, against which policy and practice should be evaluated, and developments designed.

Developments in schools have been influenced by theoretical models so that parents have had more active involvement in their children's education. Projects such as the paired reading scheme have given parents central roles that have been shown to have significant and lasting effects on children's attainment (Topping, 1986; Diaper, 1990). So, in schools as well as in therapy settings, there are examples of parents doing more than just liaising with professionals. Their participation has been sought, gained and valued.

Assimilating the Different Perspectives of Collaboration

The preceding discussion leads to an observation that therapists' views on collaboration seem to have been influenced by a range of conceptual models, whereas teachers' perspectives tend to be grounded in roles and applications in practice. There is much value in either orientation, and the first challenge for professionals collaborating together may be to try to assimilate the worthwhile aspects from both approaches.

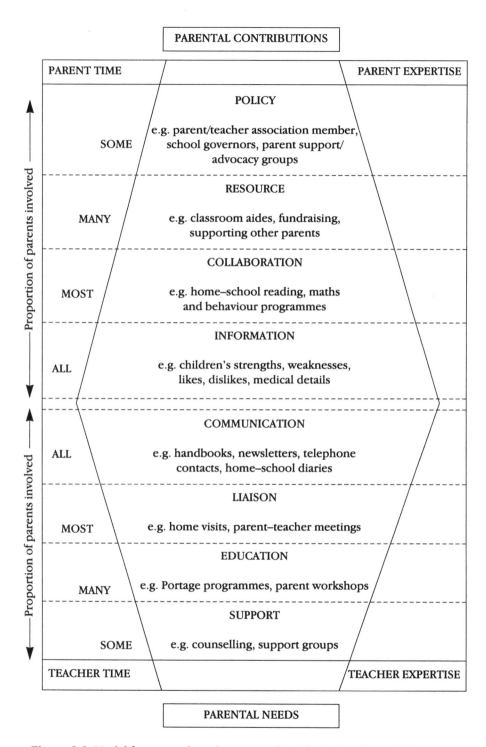

PARENTAL CONTRIBUTIONS

PARENT TIME   PARENT EXPERTISE

POLICY

SOME   e.g. parent/teacher association member, school governors, parent support/ advocacy groups

RESOURCE

MANY   e.g. classroom aides, fundraising, supporting other parents

COLLABORATION

MOST   e.g. home–school reading, maths and behaviour programmes

INFORMATION

ALL   e.g. children's strengths, weaknesses, likes, dislikes, medical details

COMMUNICATION

ALL   e.g. handbooks, newsletters, telephone contacts, home–school diaries

LIAISON

MOST   e.g. home visits, parent–teacher meetings

EDUCATION

MANY   e.g. Portage programmes, parent workshops

SUPPORT

SOME   e.g. counselling, support groups

TEACHER TIME   TEACHER EXPERTISE

PARENTAL NEEDS

Proportion of parents involved

Proportion of parents involved

Figure 8.2: Model for parental involvement with teachers, Hornby's (1995) Reproducrd from Hornby: Working with Parents of Children with Special Needs (1995) by permission of Cassell Plc, Wellington House, 125 Strand, London.

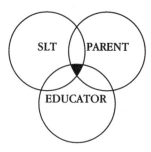

Figure 8.3: Diagram showing three-way collaboration (shaded area)

Related to this there is the practical challenge of how to accommodate a central role for parents in the developing collaborative relationship. For collaboration with parents to be integral rather than fragmented, it is necessary to forge pathways that include parents in at least a three-way consortium (such as that mapped in Figure 8.3).

It is time to move on from the various splinter approaches to parents that risk duplication and inconsistency. And it is vital to do so in a way that respects the different traditions of involving parents that have been prevalent in both SLT and teaching.

An Illustration from Practice

Figure 8.1 (p.151) showed that in practice the links between therapists and parents often co-exist alongside, but unconnected to, contact between teachers and parents. The parent in such circumstances is not integral in a three-way collaboration, but an end-point of various channels of communication. This final section aims to illustrate that point, and indicate some ways in which one service could develop to move toward the collaboration represented in Figure 8.3. The focus of this illustration is a school in central Scotland, educating children with learning disabilities.

An overview of practice in a school

Links between teaching staff and parents
Teaching staff have separate initiatives to improve their links with parents. As well as routine contact through reports, parents' evenings and daily diaries, parents have been invited to the school for workshops about new approaches to curriculum delivery. Parents have been invited to vote on matters as practical as the choice of school uniform, and have had input into devising the school code – both positive contributions to school ethos.

Links between SLTs and parents
Therapists, too, have made their own attempts to relate more closely to parents. Termly reports and attendance at parents' evenings are routine, and home visits, training and programmes for completion at home are all avail-

able. In addition, therapists host informal evenings for information and support each term. As an ongoing development, literature for parents making known the various means of therapy delivery is in preparation.

Links between parents and the school community

Parents are active in promoting advances. They have grasped opportunities to create several channels of involvement in the life of the school, including the school board, the parent/teacher association and involvement in many social and recreational activities. A small group of parents lobbied community education services to set up a club for pupils that is held in the school building. In another initiative, parents set up their own information and support group which meets in the school on a regular basis.

Links between teaching and therapy staff

In recent years, concerted efforts have been made to increase and formalise collaboration between therapists and teaching staff, as part of the school's development plan. One particular initiative has seen therapy plans being incorporated into the child's class-held forward plan and updated termly after joint discussion. In a related development, annual therapy reports are appended to the class report, in a move intended to ensure consistent communication to parents.

In all the ways that have been described, parents and professionals have been brought closer together. There are many examples of good practice, and of committed movement towards increased and better quality contact. In many ways, the school is not exceptional, and indeed there are many such developments going on quietly in schools nationally. It is important that the effort going into the moves is recognised and valued.

What has been presented is, however, a snapshot of current work. There is much more room for progress, and developments are ongoing. The connections between the three parties have been best described under separate headings, which perhaps indicates that they still exist independently of one another. That point is illustrated in the following comments from the experience of one parent involved in the system.

One parent's view

Links between teaching staff and parents

Really, all the direct contact I had with the teachers was if I had to go into the school to pick [the child] up for a hospital appointment. They would say you were allowed to come into class anytime, but I always felt I was intruding because teaching was going on. I had the diary every day, or supposed to be every day. There wasn't a lot of content in the diary anyway, just what happened in the day, just general information, nothing in-depth.

I'm a great believer that the teacher is the one who is trained. As a mother I know my child's personality, but my child is a different person when he is at school. Unless the parent has a very strong personality (which is unusual) the parent is usually led by the professional.

Links between SLTs and parents

The therapist was running a parents' evening, which was quite informative. I quite enjoyed it, meeting other parents. I think only three or four parents turned up. It was always the same core that turned up, it always is. So I felt she was banging her head against a brick wall.

I've never come up against a programme for my child that is not right. Any idea that has been brought up, as far as I am concerned, has been a good idea that I couldn't see as being detrimental in any way.

Links between parents and the school community

I went to the fundraising committees every now and again but I didn't do very much because my commitments are here at home at the moment. The only parents I had contact with were the parents I had contact with before [the child] went to school. There was never any suggestion of being friends with any other parents, I think because most were working. I'm a quiet person anyway, and if people don't live near me I don't really get to know them. There was a club for children, I think, but I didn't have anything to do with it. Apathy on my part, I suppose, and I don't know if the age group was right.

Links between teaching staff and SLTs

The therapist told me she had been in class and had told them what had to be done. But I honestly don't know how much contact there is. I don't think any parent knows. It could have been 6 months ago. It is probably pie in the sky, but I'd say once every 6 months, every 3 months, even every month is not adequate. I'd say more like once a week, though I know that can't be done.

Towards a three-way interaction of parent, teacher and therapist

The parent quoted above also commented on her perceptions of the three-way relationship:

The teacher was never involved when it was me and the speech therapist. It can't be done. The teacher can't be called out of class to be asked her opinion. In an ideal world that is exactly what would have happened but she has another six children or so to look after. I didn't think that was adequate, but you have to work within that system, don't you?

It is still a case of 'you're the teacher, you're the therapist and you're the parent'. The parent is third in line. I would say it is first the teacher, then the therapist, then the parent.

With reference to the need for three-way collaboration rather than separate links, there are ways in which this particular school could move forward. For instance, parents attending parents' evenings currently have separate audiences with the teacher and therapist. Collaboration would perhaps be more easily achieved if all three were together to jointly plan and review children's progress. Also, reports from teacher and therapist that are currently completed separately and then brought together might first be amalgamated into one joint report, and perhaps in a second development they could be dovetailed with parents' accounts of progress. In those ways, there would be more overlapping between the domains of teacher, therapist and parent in activity that would more closely resemble the collaborative core represented at the heart of Figure 8.3.

Conclusion

If collaboration with parents is to be achieved by teachers and therapists, a first hurdle may be to overcome differences in each discipline's orientation to parents. What is required is a team approach that sees parents as central members of that team. New roles will be required of all participants, calling for new knowledge, skills and attitudes. The resources needed to meet the challenge are many and varied; among them are time, money, commitment, energy, training, support, administration, policy and more. The cost, of course, is heavy. The opportunities are there, nevertheless, for a positive future of fruitful collaboration.

Chapter 9
Evaluating Efficacy

ELSPETH McCARTNEY

Introduction

Collaborative practice is in the end aiming at a 'good outcome' – an improvement in a child's ability to communicate effectively, and to learn. Teachers and SLTs are both keen to know whether this has taken place, and if so how much has been gained. There are questions beyond this about the child's quality of life during the learning process and about the efficient use of resources in achieving language and communication gains. These questions are also highly relevant to collaborative practice and deserve to be answered. SLTs and teachers are educated to be self-reflective and to evaluate their work with children on a day-to-day basis, and are keen to address such questions; and those allocating resources will also have interests in knowing they have been put to good use. However, once again health and education services have evolved in different ways, and have come to differ in the priorities they give to particular questions and the ways in which questions are asked. This chapter considers these issues, and tries to identify purposeful ways in which effectiveness can be measured in collaborative settings, using the by now familiar systems model.

Problems in Measuring Effectiveness

Practitioners concerned with evaluating effectiveness are often put off by the fact that many of the most powerful paradigms for evaluating what they do are difficult to operate in an education setting. In particular, comparative research designs that use random allocation of children to programmes are very difficult to set up. In real-life services, practitioners tend not to have control of this factor: decisions about where children are educated are based on educational and social decisions and not amenable to random allocation. Comparative research designs also favour the setting-up of carefully matched groups of children, controlling for as many relevant variables as possible. This poses a difficulty when children's complex communication and learning is under scrutiny. It is hard to find children who 'match' other children on a range of relevant variables, such as their particular language, communication and education goals, or their individual learning styles. This is particularly difficult in small-scale settings such as schools, where children with a wide range of individual goals can be present in one classroom, and where staff cannot go outside the school context to seek comparable children. Random control research designs also benefit from measurement of progress being carried out by 'blind' assessors who do not know what programme has been offered to an individual child. Practitioners are usually assessing a child's progress themselves, as well as delivering an education and therapy programme, and so cannot be 'blind' to the learning experiences offered.

There are also difficulties in evaluating the additional effects of services such as SLTs in collaborative settings. A school provides such a complex set of planned education experiences, to say nothing of adventitious experiences, that it is hard to identify one set of experiences as critical. Furthermore, it will often be impossible to develop an education or therapy package and deliver it in a predetermined way across different schools and classes. The education and social philosophy behind service delivery in the UK involves professionals adapting and using programmes as they see fit. Programmes are tailored to individual children and take account of educational opportunities as they arise. It is hard to know what can be measured in such contexts. Large-scale random control trials are designed to solve some of these problems, but as stated are often beyond the resources of individual collaborating teams.

Teachers and SLTs are keen to evaluate the total learning experiences of children, and may not need to consider the efficiency of a total package by identifying the value of separate components. Service managers, however, may be interested in trying to isolate one aspect of the whole, such as the contribution of the SLT to the process. As professional practice becomes more integrated this becomes harder to do, and probably seems less than relevant to those involved in the classroom. Any attempt to vary for example the amount or timing of SLT input in the interests of measuring efficiency would possibly be resisted, and would also come up against timetabling and other school organisational constraints.

These factors mean that many research paradigms are difficult to organise in collaborative education settings. This presents two difficulties for evaluating collaborative work. One is that staff whose model of research is based on controlled studies may recognise the problems and conclude that it is not possible to measure effectiveness at all, rather than concluding that other methods are needed. The other difficulty is that randomised control studies are seen as the 'gold standard' in health-care research (Fahey et al., 1995). Other kinds of evaluation techniques that are common in education contexts are less well developed in health settings; and although their value is becoming recognised as a means of complementing and enriching other methodologies (Pope and Mays, 1995), their acceptance remains rather limited. This can give SLTs a problem in communicating with health service decision makers.

Education evaluation, on the other hand, has long recognised the difficulties and, indeed, inappropriateness of operating traditional research designs and makes use of other kinds of methodologies. The contrast in outlook is discussed clearly by Milne (1987), who distinguishes what he calls an 'evaluative format', as used in education studies, from traditional classical approaches. He notes that, where random control studies are not possible, other types of investigation using qualitative methods can be helpful in understanding the perspectives of practitioners and in measuring changes in children. Such evaluative inquiry responds to the circumstances to which it is applied, and does not attempt to force real-life contexts into inappropriate research paradigms. Evaluative studies will give information on a local service, although results will not necessarily generalise to other contexts and will lack a measure of objectivity. Evaluative approaches must also be systematic and recognise the limits of their applicability (MacKay et al., 1996). If they can do this, they provide a useful framework for looking at the effectiveness of collaborative work, and for making decisions in small-scale education settings. The loss of the random control study is not seen as a great problem in education, and the development of collaborative practice has not come about as a result of large-scale studies comparing one type of practice with another. It has emerged from small-scale descriptive study reports and from a commitment to the principles of collaboration.

Teachers and SLTs therefore look to qualitative methods to demonstrate efficacy in collaborative settings. The most common methods employed involve a combination of 'case study' methodologies, which allow consideration of individual children's progress, and service evaluation approaches such as audit (CSLT, 1993b) and school development planning.

The Dimensions of Evaluation

Using qualitative and evaluative methods will help to answer the relevant questions about service provision and delivery, but what questions should be asked? McCartney and van der Gaag (1996) give a list of factors that an 'ideal' evaluation protocol in an education setting would have to consider, which is adapted here.

An 'ideal' evaluation protocol

An 'ideal' evaluation protocol would have to take into account:
- details of the level and organisation of services allocated to pupils – in terms of child–therapist and child–teacher contacts, staff time spent (teacher, therapist and other), and including a review of the organisational structures used to set up, deliver, evaluate and review service provision
- the perceptions of the whole school – in particular about the benefits of services
- the perceptions of parents and children – (and perhaps indirect users such as education authorities) in relation to the benefits of services
- changes in specified and predicted aspects of children's language and communication behaviours – as outcomes of education experiences, for example attainment of individual IEP goals
- the effects, if any, of targeted provision on the ongoing education progress of children
- the costs of services and the resources devoted to them.

McCartney and van der Gaag (1996: 319)

A 'good outcome' would therefore be stated in terms of services which were well received by children, parents and school staff, and which had demonstrable benefits to the child's communication development, and which had enhanced the child's educational attainments. Measuring this would involve collecting different types of evidence. Much of this evidence would be collected in any case as an integral part of routine working practices, gathered as part of IEP and review procedures. Additional data would be needed on child, parent and staff perceptions of service. Such a route to evaluating effectiveness can capture the real-life complexities of collaborative working.

A Coordinating Systems Framework

Once again, the systems framework used throughout this book can be used to provide a coordinating framework within which to evaluate efficacy. McCartney and van der Gaag (1996) outline ways in which this approach can be used. There is a need to ensure that information is shared across services at all levels, and managerial decisions will need to be made on how this is to be done.

Function measures

Function measures are central to measures of efficacy, answering questions about whether a collaborative approach is meeting its overall aim of helping children to communicate. The ability to answer the question 'How will we know if we have helped?' depends on a clear idea of what was being aimed for, both in terms of child gains and in attaining 'good' collaborative practice. There needs to be an overall statement of policies: what was being attempted and what would constitute a good picture of a good outcome. For children's progress there will be measures of goals attained to be extracted from their IEP. Measures of collaborative practice can be extracted from structures such as service-level agreements and functions like prioritisation procedures. These feed back into the process of evaluating efficacy. Questions about collaboration which can be answered from such documents include the following:

Function questions about collaboration

- did the planned contacts between teachers and SLTs to discuss and exchange information take place?
- were the planned number of joint inservice sessions carried out?
- did the SLT attend the school as planned?
- were joint aims constructed for individual children?
- were joint records kept?
- who consulted records, and did they find them helpful?
- did the child access the differentiated curriculum as planned?
- were most children reaching their goals?

Some information can be obtained from professionals' logs, diaries and reports, and from children's attendance records. It is sensible to maintain a database that allows such contacts to be monitored and collated. Similarly, children's timetables can be used to look at the ways in which children, teachers and SLTs have met to work on a differentiated curriculum for the child, and classroom records will be useful. There may also be specific therapy time, and access to a learning support teacher or classroom assistant, which should be recorded.

Such measures are largely quantitative, and check what actually happened against agreed service-level plans. They are also useful as a basis for discussion to monitor functions in general. Many things can get in the way of delivering an agreed plan, and service-level plans can be reviewed in light of such information. Issues around different models of selecting children and assessing need, the social interaction of professionals and the sharing of professional information can also be discussed as part of this review, to further clarify roles and expectations of collaboration.

The second important strand of measuring functional efficacy is to evaluate the progress made by children receiving services. This information is gained from the children's IEPs, where goals are logged and communication aims listed. There are also standard curriculum attainments which may be useful but which may not be sufficiently sensitive to measure limited progress, and may not cover child-specific aims (Mason, 1994). Children who are making progress towards their planned aims would be seen as having benefited in most collaborative programmes, and most parents would be happy with such information. However, in SLT services and for some service allocation purposes it is sometimes considered useful to assess the progress of children as compared with something else – usually against the amount of change that might have been expected from normally developing children without language and communication difficulties and without specific intervention. In this context, standardised or developmental assessments are often used to measure language gains (McCartney, 1993).

Function measures and process measures

Individual child attainment measures (sometimes referred to as 'outcome' measures) from IEP goals will feed into evaluation at two levels. They can help to evaluate the education process, where an individual child's progress and interaction with the collaborative system is evaluated. They also feed into evaluations of function, where a service is evaluating how well it is achieving its aims. A service should seek to aggregate measures of how individual children are achieving their goals and to summate these into a measure of how well the service is functioning in its aim of helping children. A straightforward list is helpful, and in view of the complexities involved and the difficulties of comparison may be the best measure. More formal approaches to service evaluation do exist, such as Goal Attainment Scaling, which is designed to summate the progress of a variety of children with a variety of educational aims and outcomes (MacKay et al., 1993b, 1996). Such approaches may be useful to measure success across a range of classroom settings.

Structure measures

Structure measures give an account of services' organisational structures and their decision-making procedures. They consider managerial and staff groupings, and the structured ways in which opinion is sought by the service. They include notes of fairly permanent features of a service such as the school year, timetables, managerial organisation (such as who reports to whom), and how information is passed around the system. There is usually a need to share information of this type between services, and to update it regularly.

Questions to be answered include the following:

Structure questions

- who allocates SLT input?
- who allocates teacher time for collaboration?
- how do services join to take decisions on such matters:
    at a national or regional level?
    at a trust and education authority level?
    at an SLT service manager and headteacher level?
    at a class and support teacher and SLT level?

- how are joint decisions recorded?
- who tells who what, and when?
- how are others, such as parents, brought into the decision-making process?

Measures here are largely descriptive, and fairly easy to obtain by consulting relevant policy documents and by discussion. It is, however, important to share information across services, and this is an area where difficulties have arisen in the past. Clarifying decision-making procedures and constraints is an important part of collaborative working.

Process measures

Process measures track the event sequence concerned with a child's contact with a service – entry to it, interaction within it and leaving it. Most of the information is usually contained in a child's records, and relates to a particular individual. Measures of attainment from IEPs also help to measure success.

There is also a need to consider the overall workings of the collaborative system; such as pre-school assessment team meetings, the defining and listing of a child's special education needs to whatever stage of formal statementing or recording, and the regular review of these needs. There is detailed guidance on these aspects in the code of practice (DfE, 1994, 1999) and in the Scottish EPSEN document (SOEID, 1994). SLT services collect similar information as part of audit processes, and of course information must once again be shared. Process questions to be answered include the following:

Process questions

- are services meeting national good practice standards –
    concerning listing and reviewing a child's language and special needs?
    concerning clinical audit procedures?
- are services taking child perspectives into account?
- are services taking staff perspectives into account?
- are individual children attaining their IEP and language goals?

Measures here are descriptive, and might employ questionnaire and interview techniques. In addition, children's goals attained from IEPs and language gains from standardised and criterion-referenced assessments can be considered.

Systems-environment measures

Systems-environment measures consider the context in which a service operates. Throughout this book the importance of parents has been stressed, and the ways in which they can be involved in collaborative work, although there are many other aspects of context that are also relevant. The notion of 'good practice' has to be related to the rapidly developing knowledge base concerned with children with language and communication difficulties, and charitable bodies such as the Association for all Speech Impaired Children (AFASIC) and the National Association of Special Education Needs (NASEN) give useful guidance and information. There is also a need to feed back to the systems environment information on good collaborative practice which is taking place, and the limits placed upon it, and the ways in which development could be aided. Questions relevant to the environment include the following:

Systems enviroment questions

- are services informing relevant bodies in the local environment about practices?
- are services meeting the needs of parents?
- are services employing up-to-date practices?
- are services meeting good practice guidelines in general?
- are services explaining their constraints and seeking help to develop?

Methods of answering such questions include holding meetings and organised discussions, and using questionnaires, reports and presentations. Information is significantly easier to obtain if good interaction pertains at a functional level, and if structures are in place to access the relevant people in the systems environment.

The Use of the Coordinating Framework

The measures needed to get a 'good fix' on services are not extensive, and can mostly be gathered as part of the routine information-gathering procedures common in most services. There are a few commercial databases that can deal with some of the issues (SiLAS, 1993), but further development of software to help record collaborative practice is needed. The questions to be asked are not new, but the systems approach may help to give practitioners confidence that their measures of effectiveness are those best adapted to answer the real-life questions posed in real-life contexts. An illustration from practice might help.

A systems approach to evaluation of efficacy

Liddell (1997) used a systems approach to consider the collaborative services offered to three children (coded A, B and C) with Asperger's syndrome.

Systems environment
All three children received input from one SLT service based in an NHS trust. SLT provision in school was partly funded by the children's education authority. The SLT worked to RCSLT professional guidelines advocating collaborative

working. The duration of SLT input had been two school terms. To this extent, the background environmental and contextual features within which collaboration took place were the same.

Child A	Child B	Child C
Structure measures		
Aged 8 years. Attends mainstream primary school.	Aged 9 years. Attends a special communication disorders unit located in a mainstream primary school, with minimal integration with mainstream peers at this stage.	Aged 8 years. Attends mainstream primary school.
Class teacher holds no special qualification in special needs or communication disorder. Assistant headteacher in role of special education needs coordinator.	A specialist teacher qualified in communication disorders at masters level is available.	No additional support in class.
SLT operates an open, informal communication system in school.	SLT time allocation is two sessions a week to six children.	SLT contact in class and one-to-one with child once monthly. Additional SLT regular sessions in home setting. No formal documentation of service structure established to date.
No school service level agreement at present.	Written school service level agreement.	No dedicated SLT and teacher contact time. School feels this is not practical.
Function measures		
No mutual evaluation system devised in relation to communication goals set – progress recorded by informal perception measures.	Joint recording of goals and programme details by class teacher and SLT.	SLT devised communication programme. No mutual evaluation system for communication goals agreed.

Child A	Child B	Child C
No quantitative outcome measures available as yet. SLT monitors programme and child's communication progress in monthly session in class.	Quantitative scoring system used to evaluate all goals, including communication goals.	
SLT devised training programme for teachers	Timetable of training sessions implemented jointly by specialist teacher and SLT and delivered separately to teachers and parents group.	SLT implementing a programme of whole team meetings in school.
Regular review meetings involve parent, school team and educational psychologist.	Regular review and planning meetings in school.	Review meetings held in response to parental request.

Process measures

No record of needs as yet.	Child has record of needs.	Child following class curriculum.
Detailed IEP devised jointly between SLT and teacher following 5–14 Curriculum.	Individual IEP devised jointly by SLT, class teacher, specialist teacher and parents.	No IEP as yet. Teacher reports great difficulties implementing SLT programme without increased support and contact with SLT.
Teacher interviews report increase in communication skills and increased satisfaction with SLT services.	Quantitative measures from IEP indicate good progress.	Teacher interviews reveal limited progress to date.

Systems-environment measures

Parent interviews report increase in communication skills and increased satisfaction with SLT services.	Parental questionnaires devised by SLT and school indicate overall parental satisfaction with collaborative service.	Parental interviews reveal limited progress to date. Liddell (1997)

Liddell (1997) comments that the systems approach proved useful in documenting the diversity of levels of collaboration achieved in one locality, as the example above shows. She suggests that such approaches could lead to a quantitative scoring procedure but notes that even descriptive analyses offer specific insights to key areas of strength and weakness operating in each case. For child C, where collaboration is minimal, the SLT service needs to provide a definite statement of SLT expectations, and to both inform the school and engage it in a more collaborative education approach for this child. A school-level service agreement may serve this purpose. She also notes a need for SLT input to train staff and increase the school's awareness of need and to stress the value of working together to meet the child's communication, social and overall education needs. The systems evaluation also shows that, for children A and B, the SLT service offered differs on variables of time allocation, school staff expertise and opportunities for mainstream integration. However, in spite of these variables, the early measures of people's perception of the service showed a positive response to the collaborative working model. Liddell concludes that the systems approach:

> has much to offer and has, even in this limited form, provided a fruitful basis on which to develop evaluation mechanisms needed to measure client gain and service efficacy even more efficiently in the future. Use of an evaluation model has the added benefit of being universally understood by all involved in the collaborative working model (p. 6).

Practical utility will be the test of such an approach, but there seems to be a place for a coordinating framework to structure evaluation approaches in collaborative settings. The systems model adopted has potential in this context, and provides a set of useful questions that staff might employ in considering the effectiveness of intervention.

Conclusion

This book reflects a point in time when it seems possible to look forward to collaborative working becoming the normal and expected means by which education and SLT services are delivered to school children. The overall impression gained from reviewing the field is that it is the SLT profession that has made the most change, by giving up its 'expert who extracts' role and moving to the classroom. SLTs may have taken education services somewhat by surprise in the process, and are now rapidly forming decision-making bodies and developing policy statements and explanatory documents to detail what is going on. Education is broadly welcoming of such initiatives, but may have to move a little further in making the SLTs feel entirely welcome. Education as a system is somewhat unused to dealing with professionals who expect to be partners who collaborate rather than employees to be controlled. Once again, however, the education system is adapting to accommodate change, and capitalising fast on partnership opportunities. New structures that allow sensible joint planning are emerging, and are expected to develop rapidly.

A broad systems analysis shows that there are still a number of barriers to be overcome to achieve good collaboration, and in particular the issues of the amount of SLT input required to deliver an adequate service and the funding of SLT services to schools stand out as requiring resolution. There are particular difficulties in mainstream schools. At all systems levels, however, it proved possible to find examples of good collaborative practice, although many of these came from small-scale studies and reflected local solutions to particular problems. It is hoped that collating such examples and organising them in one coordinating framework will prove helpful to practitioners seeking to make sense of their own context, and will encourage the creation and dissemination of further instances. There is certainly a need for many more illustrations of good practice, and for much further interprofessional discussion of ways in which progress can be made. This book has concentrated on two professions only, and consideration of the perspectives of a number of others is also needed. As far as teachers and SLTs are concerned, however, their commitment to collaboration suggests an encouraging future.

References

AFASIC (1990) *Education Facilities Available for Communication Impaired Children*. London: Association for All Speech Impaired Children.

AFASIC (1993) *Speech and Language Therapy as Educational Provision – A Guide to the Present State of the Law on SLT for Children of School Age*. London: Association for All Speech Impaired Children.

AFASIC (1997) Speech and language therapy – 'No let out' for LEAs. *AFASIC Newsletter* 1997: 4. London: Association for All Speech Impaired Children.

Anderson, H., Graham, F., Constable, A. (1990) *Activities for Speaking, Listening and Confidence in Communicating*. London: Association for All Speech Impaired Children.

Andrews, G., Craig, A., Feyer, A., Hoddinott, S., Howie, P., Neilson, M. (1983) Stuttering: A review of research findings and theories circa 1982. *Journal of Speech and Hearing Disorders* 48: 226–46.

Apple, M.W. (1993) *Official Knowledge*. London: Routledge.

Appleton, P.L., Minchom, P.E. (1990) Models of Parent Partnership and Child Development Centres. Department of Paediatrics, Wrexham Maelor Hospital, Clwyd Health Authority, Wrexham, Clwyd, Wales.

Atkin, J., Bastiani, J. (1988) Training teachers to work with parents. In Bastiani, J. (Ed.) *Parents and Teachers 2: From Policy to Practice*. Windsor: NFER.

Attwood, T. (1998) *Asperger's Syndrome*. London: Jessica Kingsley.

Banathy, B. (1973) *Developing a Systems View of Education*. Belmont: Siegler.

Banathy, B. (1991) *Systems Design of Education: A Journey to Create the Future*. Englewood Cliffs, NJ: Educational Technology Publications.

Banathy, B. (1992) *A Systems View of Education: Concepts and Principles for Effective Practice*. Englewood Cliffs, NJ: Educational Technology Publications.

Banathy, B. (1996) *Designing Social Systems in a Changing World*. New York: Plenum Press.

Barnett, P., Fletcher-Wood, V. (1983) *Let's Play Language*. Wisbech: Learning Development Aids.

Bastiani, J. (1989) *Working with Parents : A Whole-school Approach*. Windsor: NFER.

Beazley, S., Moore, M. (1995) *Deaf Children, Their Families and Professionals: Dismantling Barriers*. London: David Fulton.

Beck, A.R., Dennis, M. (1997) Speech-language pathologists' and teachers' perceptions of classroom-based interventions. *Language, Speech and Hearing Services in Schools*, **28**, 146–52.

Bedrosian, J. (1985) An approach to developing conversational competence. In Ripich, D., Spinelli, F. (Eds) *School Discourse Problems*. San Diego, CA: College Hill Press, pp. 239–40

Bell, R.Q. (1968) A reinterpretation of the direction of effects in studies of socialisation. *Psychological Review*, **75**: 81–95.

Bicknell, J. (1988) The psychopathology of handicap In Horobin, G., May, D. (Eds) *Living with Mental Handicap: Transitions in the Lives of People with Mental Handicaps*. London: Jessica Kingsley, pp. 22–37.

Bishop, D.V.M., Edmundson, A. (1987) Language-impaired 4-year-olds: distinguishing transient from persistent impairment. *Journal of Speech and Hearing Disorders*, **51**: 98–110.

Bloodstein, O. (1995) *A Handbook on Stuttering*. London: Singular.

Bothwell, A. (1997) Establishing a Collaborative Partnership Between the Speech and Language Therapy Service and the Education Department in a Mainstream School Setting. Submitted in part-fulfilment of postgraduate award, Department of Speech and Language Therapy, University of Strathclyde.

British Stammering Association (1995) *Bullying and the Dysfluent Child in Primary School*. London: British Stammering Association.

British Stammering Association (1996) *A Chance to Speak*. London: British Stammering Association.

Bronfenbrenner, U. (1979) *The Ecology of Human Development*. Cambridge, MA: Harvard University Press.

Bryce, T. (1993) Challenges to the management of assessment. In Humes, W., MacKenzie, M. (Eds) *The Management of Education Policy; Scottish Perspectives*. London: Longman, pp. 31–51.

Burnell, M., Harkness, S. (1992) Each, Peach, Pear, Plum. In Ahlberg, J. and Ahlberg, A.: *A Picture Story Book Study Guide*. Harlow: Oliver & Boyd.

Charter, D. (1997) The speaking window of opportunity. *The Times*, **30 May**: 39.

Conoley, J.C., Conoley, C.W. (1982) *School Consultation: A Guide to Practice and Training*. Oxford: Pergamon.

Conti-Ramsden, G., Donlan, C., Grove, J. (1992) Children with specific language impairments: Curricular opportunities and school performance. *British Journal of Special Education*, **19**: 75–80.

Cooper, E.B. (1975) Clinician Attitudes Toward Stutterers: A Study of Bigotry? Paper presented at the Convention of the American Speech and Hearing Association, Washington, DC.

Cooper, E., Cooper, C. (1985) Clinician attitudes towards stuttering: A decade of change (1973–1983). *Journal of Fluency Disorders*, **10**: 19–33.

Cooper, E., Rustin, L. (1985) Clinician attitudes toward stuttering in the United States and Great Britain: A cross cultural study. *Journal of Fluency Disorders*, **10**: 1–17.

Crais, E.R. (1991) Moving from parent involvement to family-centred services. *American Journal of Speech and Language Therapy*, 5–8

Crowe, T., Walton, J. (1981) Teacher attitudes towards stuttering. *Journal of Fluency Disorders*, **6**: 163–74.

CSLT (1993a) Speech and language therapy in education. Bulletin, College of Speech and Language Therapists, **July**: 7–8.

CSLT (1993b) *Audit: A Manual for Speech and Language Therapists*. London: College of Speech and Language Therapists.

Cunningham, C., Davis, H. (1985) *Working with Parents: Frameworks for Collaboration*. Buckingham: Open University Press.

Daines, B. (1992) Crossing the divide: The relationship between teaching in class and speech and language therapy programme objectives. In Miller, C. (Ed.) *The Education System and Speech Therapy: Proceedings of an AFASIC Conference*. London: City University, pp. 15–23.

Daines, B., Fleming, P., Miller, C. (1996) *Speech and Language Difficulties: Spotlight on Special Education Needs*. Tamworth: National Association for Special Education Needs.

Dale, P.S., Cole, K.N. (1991) What's normal? Specific language impairment in an individual differences perspective. *Language, Speech and Hearing Services in Schools*, 22: 80–3.

Dalton, P., Hardcastle, W. (1977) *Disorders of Fluency*. London: Arnold.

David, R., Smith, B. (1987) Preparing for collaborative working. *British Journal of Special Education*, 14: 19–23.

David, R., Smith, B. (1991) Collaboration in initial training. In Upton, G. (Ed.) *Staff Training and Special Education Needs*. London: David Fulton, pp. 102–9.

Davidson, F.M., Howlin, P. (1997) A follow up study of children attending a primary-age language unit. *European Journal of Disorders of Communication*, 32: 19–36.

Davie, R. (1993) Implementing Warnock's multidisciplinary approach. In Visser, J., Upton, G. (Eds) *Special Education in Britain after Warnock*. London: David Fulton, pp. 138–50.

De Lamerens-Pratt, M., Golden, G.S. (1994) Teamwork in medical settings – Hospitals, clinics and communities. In Garner, H.G., Orelove, F.P. (Eds) *Teamwork in Human Services*. Newton: Butterworth-Heinemann, pp. 159–77.

DES (1975) *A Language for Life (The Bullock Report)*. London: HMSO.

DES (1978) *Special Educational Needs, the 'Warnock Report'*. London: HMSO.

DES (1989) *National Curriculum from Policy to Practice*. London: HMSO.

Dessent, T. (1996) *Meeting Special Educational Needs – Options for Partnership Between Health, Social and Educational Services*. Tamworth: National Association for Special Educational Needs.

DfE (1994) *The Code of Practice on the Identification and Assessment of Special Educational Needs*. London: Department for Education.

DfEE (1997) *Excellence for All Children*. London: Stationery Office.

DfEE (1998) Meeting Special Educational Needs: A Programme of Action. London: Department for Education and the Environment.

DfEE (1999) The SEN Code of Practice and Associated Legislation – Proposed Changes and Areas for Revision. London: Department for Education and the Environment.

Diaper, G. (1990) A comparative study of paired-reading techniques using parents as tutors to second-year junior school children. *Child Language Teaching and Therapy*, 6: 13–24.

DiMeo, J.H., Merritt, D.D., Culatta, B. (1998) Collaborative partnerships and decision making. In Merritt, D., Culatta, B. (Eds) *Language Intervention in the Classroom*. San Diego: Singular, pp. 37–96.

DoH (1989) *Working for Patients*. London: Department of Health.

DoH (1992) *The Health of the Nation*. London: HMSO.

DoH (1998) Partnership in Action – New Opportunities for Joint Working between Health and Social Services. London: Department of Health.

Donaldson, M.L. (1995) *Children with Language Impairments*. London: Jessica Kingsley.

Dunst, C.J., Trivette, C., Deal, A. (1988) *Enabling and Empowering Families*. Cambridge, MA: Brookline.

Elksnin, L.K., Capilouto, G.J. (1994) Speech and language pathologists' perceptions of integrated service delivery in school settings. *Language, Speech and Hearing Services in Schools*, 25: 258–68.

Emblem, B., Conti-Ramsden, G. (1990) Towards level 1: Reality or illusion? *British Journal of Special Education*, 17: 88–90.

Enderby, P., Davies, P. (1989) Communication disorders: Planning a service to meet the needs. *British Journal of Disorders of Communication*, **21**: 151–66.

Fahey, T., Griffiths, S., Peters, T. (1995) Evidence based purchasing: Understanding the results of clinical trials and systematic reviews. *British Medical Journal*, **311**: 1056–60.

Fourali, C. (1997) Using fuzzy logic in education assessment: The case of portfolio assessment. *Evaluation and Research in Education*, **11**: 129–48.

Gains, C., Smith, C. (1994) Cluster models. *Support for Learning*, **9**: 94–8.

Gargiulo, R.M. (1985) *Working with Parents of Exceptional Children: A Guide for Professionals*. Boston: Houghton Mifflin.

Gascoigne, E. (1995) *Working with Parents as Partners in SEN*. London: David Fulton.

Gillon, G., Dodd, B. (1997) Enhancing the phonological processing skills of children with specific reading disability. *European Journal of Disorders of Communication*, **32**: 67–90.

Girolametto, L.E., Greenberg, J., Manolson, H.A. (1986) Developing dialogue skills: The Hanen Early Language Parent Programme. *Seminars in Speech and Language*, **7**: 367–82.

Girolametto, L.E., Tannock, R., Siegel, L. (1993) Consumer-oriented evaluation of interactive language intervention. *American Journal of Speech-Language Pathology*, **41**–51.

Gorrie, B., Edwards, A., McKiernan, A. (1998) Literacy: To treat or not to treat? *Bulletin of the Royal College of Speech and Language Therapists*, **May**: 9–11.

Gottwald, S., Goldbach, P., Isack, A. (1985) Stuttering Prevention and Detection. *Young Children*: 9–14.

Haggarty, P. (1997) Establishing a Collaborative Speech and Language Therapy Service. Submitted in part-fulfilment of postgraduate award, Department of Speech and Language Therapy, University of Strathclyde.

Hansard (1994) House of Lords Official Report 9th May 1994. London: HMSO.

Hayhow, R. (1995) Working with young children. In Fawcus, M. (Ed.) *Stuttering from Theory to Practice*. London: Whurr, pp. 22–43.

Hewett, B. (1986) *Compare Bears*. Wisbech: Learning Development Aids.

HMI (1978) *Pupils with Learning Difficulties in Primary and Secondary Schools in Scotland*. Edinburgh: Scottish Education Department.

HMI (1996) *The Education of Pupils with Language and Communication Disorders*. Edinburgh: The Scottish Office Education and Industry Department and HMSO.

Honeyfield, J. (1997a) 'Is this Speech Therapy?': Improving Collaboration Through Explicating Roles. Submitted in part-fulfilment of postgraduate award, Department of Speech and Language Therapy, University of Strathclyde.

Honeyfield, J. (1997b) Developing Aims Compatible with the 5–14 Curriculum. Guidelines for a Child with Difficulties Listening and Using Language Effectively. Submitted in part-fulfilment of postgraduate award, Department of Speech and Language Therapy, University of Strathclyde.

Hornby, G. (1994) *Counselling in Child Disability*. London: Chapman and Hall.

Hornby, G. (1995) *Working with Parents of Children with Special Needs*. London: Cassell.

Horsley, I., Fitzgibbon, C. (1987) Stuttering children: investigation of a stereotype. *British Journal of Disorders of Communication*, **22**: 19–35.

Jeans, V., Seddon, C., Semple, K., Slater, G. (1997) Mainstream schools – Do they love us? *Bulletin, Royal College of Speech and Language Therapists*, **August**: 10–12.

Jordan, R., Jones, G. (1997) *Education Provision for Children with Autism in Scotland*. Interchange No. 46. Edinburgh: Scottish Office Education and Industry Department.

Kersner, M. (1996) Working together for children with severe learning disabilities. *Child Language, Teaching and Therapy*, **12**: 17–28.

Kersner, M., Wright, J. (1996) Collaboration between teachers and speech and language therapists working with severe learning disabilities (SLD): Implications for professional development. *British Journal of Learning Disabilities*, 24: 33–7.

Knowles, W., Masidlover, M. (1982) *The Derbyshire Language Scheme*. Ripley, Derbyshire. Unpublished.

Kroth, R.L. (1985) *Communicating with Parents of Exceptional Children*. Denver, CO: Love.

Kubler-Ross, E. (1969) *On Death and Dying*. New York: Macmillan.

Kugel, R., Wolfensberger, W. (Eds) (1969) *Changing Patterns in Residential Services for the Mentally Retarded*. Washington, DC: President's Commission on Mental Retardation.

LaBlance, G., Steckol, K., Smith, V. (1994) Stuttering: The role of the classroom teacher. *Teaching Exceptional Children*, **26**: 10–12.

Lacey, P. (1995) In the front line: Special education needs co-ordinators and liaison. *Support for Learning*, **10**: 57–62.

Lacey, P., Ranson, S. (1994) Partnership for learning. *Support for Learning*, **9**: 79–82.

Lass, N., Ruscello, D., Schmitt, J., Pannbacker, M., Orlando, M., Dean, K., Ruziska, J., Bradshaw, K. (1992) Teachers' perceptions of stutterers. *Language, Speech and Hearing Services in Schools*, **23**: 78–81.

Lass, N., Ruscello, D., Pannbacker, M., Schmitt, J., Kiser, A., Mussa, A., Lockhart, P. (1994) School administrators' perceptions of people who stutter. *Language, Speech and Hearing Services in Schools*, **25**: 90–3.

Law, J. (1997) Evaluating intervention for language impaired children: A review of the literature. *European Journal of Disorders of Communication*, **32**: 1–14.

Law, J., Boyle, J., Harris, F., Harkness, A., Nye, C. (1998) *Child Health Surveillance – Screening for Speech and Language Delay*. Effective Health Care Bulletins Vol. 4. Southampton: Co-ordinating Centre for Health Technology Assessment.

Lees, J., Urwin, S. (1997) *Children with Language Disorders*. London: Whurr.

Lennox, N., Watkins, K (1998) Teaching and learning together. *Bulletin, Royal College of Speech and Language Therapists*, **March**: 13–15.

Leonard, L.B. (1991) Specific language impairment as a clinical category. *Language, Speech and Hearing Services in Schools*, **22**: 66–8.

Liddell, P. (1997) Collaboration in the Education of Young People with Asperger's Syndrome: Collected Case Studies. Submitted in part-fulfilment of postgraduate award, Department of Speech and Language Therapy, University of Strathclyde.

Lindquist, E.F., Hieronymous, A.N. (1964) *Manual for Administrators, Supervisors and Counsellors, Iowa Tests of Basic Skills*. Boston, MA: Houghton Mifflin.

Lloyd, G., Ainsworth, S. (1954) The classroom teacher's activities and attitudes relating to speech correction. *Journal of Speech and Hearing Disorders*, **19**: 244–9.

Lloyd, S. (1992) *Jolly Phonics*. Essex: Jolly Learning.

Lombana, J.H. (1983) *Home–school Partnerships: Guidelines and Strategies for Educators*. New York: Grune & Stratton.

Louko, L., Edwards, M.L., Conture, E.G. (1990) Phonological characteristics of young stutterers and their normally fluent peers: Preliminary observations. *Journal of Fluency Disorders*, **15**: 191–210.

Lovey, J. (1996) Concepts in identifying effective classroom support. *Support for Learning*, **11**: 9–12.

Luscombe, M., Shaw, L. (1996) Agreeing priorities for a school service. *Bulletin, Royal College of Speech and Language Therapists*, **December**: 8–9.

McAllister, A.H. (1937) *Clinical Studies in Speech Therapy*. London: University of London Press.

McCartney, E. (1993) Assessment of expressive language. In Beech, J.R., Harding, L. (Eds) *Assessment in Speech and Language Therapy*. London: Routledge, pp. 35–48.

McCartney, E. (1996) The Glasgow School of Speech Therapy. In Harrison, M.M., Marker, W.B. (Eds) *Teaching the Teachers – a History of Jordanhill College of Education 1828–1993*. Edinburgh: John Donald, pp. 158–68

McCartney, E. (1999) Scoping and hoping. British Journal of Special; Education, 26. In press.

McCartney, E., Wilson, S. (1994) Early literacy and children with severe speech and physical impairment: A review. *European Journal of Special Needs Education*, 9: 200–14.

McCartney, E., van der Gaag, A. (1996) How shall we be judged? Speech and language therapists in educational settings. *Child Language, Teaching and Therapy*, 12: 314–27.

McCartney, E., MacKay, G., Cheseldine, S., McCool, S. (1998) The development of a systems analysis approach to small-scale education evaluation. *Educational Review*, 50: 65–73.

McCaughey, R. (1997a) Compare and Contrast the Medical Model of Multidisciplinary Working Practices with the Education Model of Collaboration. Submitted in part-fulfilment of postgraduate award, Department of Speech and Language Therapy, University of Strathclyde.

McCaughey, R. (1997b) Parents' Perspective of Services from a Child Development Centre and a Language Development Unit. Submitted in part-fulfilment of postgraduate award, Department of Speech and Language Therapy, University of Strathclyde.

McConachie, H. (1994) Changes in family roles. In Mittler, P., Mittler, H. (Eds) *Innovations in Family Support for People with Learning Disabilities*. Chorley: Lisieux Hall.

MacDonald, A., Rendle, C. (1994) Developing the foundations of communicative competence in children with severe physical disability. In Watson, J. (Ed.) *Working with Communication Difficulties*. Edinburgh: Moray House, pp. 70–87.

McGrath, J.R., Davis, A. (1992) Rehabilitation: Where are we going and how do we get there? *Clinical Rehabilitation*, 6: 225–35.

MacKay, G. (1993) Not all of the children, all of the time. *Special Children*, 69: 18–19.

MacKay, G., Lundie, J. (1998) GAS released again: Proposals for the development of goal-attainment-scaling. *International Journal of Disability, Development and Education*, 45(2): 217–31.

MacKay, G., McLarty, M. (1999). Pupils with special education needs. In Bryce, T., Humes, W. (Eds) *Education in Scotland*. Edinburgh: Edinburgh University Press, pp. 795–804.

MacKay, G., McCartney, E., McCool, S., Cheseldine, S. (1993) Conducting evaluations. *Education in the North*, 1: 37–45.

MacKay, G., McCool, S., McCartney, E., Cheseldine, S. (1993b) Goal attainment scaling: a technique for evaluating conductive education. British Journal of Special Education, 20: 143–7.

MacKay, G., McCartney, E., McCool, S., Cheseldine, S. (1995) Our little system has its day. *Proceedings of the Scottish Education Research Association*, October 1994: 91–3.

MacKay, G., McCartney, E., Cheseldine, S., McCool, S. (1996) Evaluation of the Scottish Centre for Children with Motor Impairments (the Craighalbert Centre):

Final report to the Scottish Office Education Department. Glasgow: Faculty of Education, University of Strathclyde.

MacKay, G., Anderson, C., Baldry, H., Clark, K. (1997) Education provision for children with disorders of language and communication in West Central Scotland. *Scottish Educational Review*, 29: 154–62.

Mackey, S., McQueen, J. (1998) Exploring the association between integrated therapy and inclusive education. *British Journal of Special Education*, 25: 22–7.

MacKinnon, K. (1997) The Development and Application of a Collaborative Working Framework within a Language Unit. Submitted in part-fulfilment of postgraduate award, Department of Speech and Language Therapy, University of Strathclyde.

Manning, W. (1996) *Clinical Decision Making in the Diagnosis and Treatment of Fluency Disorders*. London: Delmar.

Martin, D., Miller, C. (1996) *Speech and Language Difficulties in the Classroom*. London: David Fulton.

Marvin, C. (1990) Problems in school-based language and collaboration services: Defining the terms and improving the process. *Language, Speech and Hearing Services in Schools*, 25: 258–68.

Mason, M. (1994) Implementing language use 5–14. In Watson, J. (Ed.) *Working with Communication Difficulties*. Edinburgh: Moray House, pp. 88–105.

Mays, N., Pope, C. (1997) *Speech and Language Therapy Services and Management in the Internal Market*. London: Kings Fund.

Meikle, M.S. (1996) Priorities, Protocols and Outcomes: Contracting for your Caseload. In Proceedings of the Golden Jubilee Conference, York, 1995, pp. 85-99. London: Royal College of Speech and Language Therapists.

Merritt, D., Culatta, B. (1998) *Language Intervention in the Classroom*. San Diego, CA: Singular.

Michael, B., Michael, M. (1987) *Foundations of Language*. Glasgow: Jordanhill College.

Millar, S., Reid, J. (1996) The role of SLTs in education. *Bulletin, Royal College of Speech and Language Therapists*, **November**: 12–13.

Miller, C. (1991) The needs of teachers of children with speech and language disorders. *Child Language, Teaching and Therapy*, 7: 179–91.

Miller, C. (1994) Speech and language therapy: Confusion in the code. *British Journal of Special Education*, 21: 53–5.

Milne, D. (Ed.) (1987) *Evaluating Mental Health Practice: Methods and Applications*. New York: Croom Helm.

Mink, I.T., Nihira, K. (1987) Direction of effects: Family life styles and behaviour of TMR children. *American Journal of Mental Deficiency*, 92: 57–64.

MoE (1945) Statutory Rules and Orders No. 1076. The Handicapped Pupils and School Health Service Regulations. London: HMSO.

Montgomery, G. (1998) Letter from the chair. *Bulletin, Royal College of Speech and Language Therapists*, **June**: 2.

Mooney, S., Smith, P. (1995) Bullying and the child who stammers. *British Journal of Special Education*, 22: 24–7.

Morgan, S.R. (1985) *Children in Crisis: A Team Approach in the Schools*. London: Taylor and Francis.

NCC (1993) *Special Needs and The National Curriculum: Opportunity and Challenge*. York: National Curriculum Council.

Nippold, M. (1990) Concomitant speech and language disorders in stuttering children: A critique of the literature. *Journal of Speech and Hearing Disorders*, **55**: 51–60.

Nippold, M., Schwarz, I. (1990) Reading disorders in stuttering children. *Journal of Fluency Disorders*, **15**: 175–89.

Norwich, B. (1996) Special needs education or education for all: Connective specialism and ideological impurity. *British Journal of Special Education*, **23**: 100–4.

OUP (1986) *The Oxford Reading Tree*. Oxford: OUP.

Paul, R., Murray, C., Clancy, K., Andrews, D. (1997) Reading and metaphonological outcomes in late talkers. *Journal of Speech and Hearing Research*, **40**: 1037–47.

Peacey, N. (1992) The national curriculum and special educational needs with particular reference to speech and language difficulties. In Miller, C. (Ed.) *The Education System and Speech Therapy: Proceedings of an AFASIC Conference*. London: City University.

Peters, T., Guitar, B. (1991) *Stuttering: An Integrated Approach to its Nature and Treatment*. London: Williams & Wilkins.

Pindzola, R. (1985) Classroom teachers; interacting with stutterers. *Teacher Education*, **21**: 2–8.

Pope, C., Mays, N. (1995) Researching the parts other methods cannot reach: An introduction to qualitative methods in health and health services research. *British Medical Journal*, **311**: 42–5.

Popple, J., Wellington, W. (1996) Collaborative working within a psycholinguistic framework. *Child Language Teaching and Therapy*, **12**: 60–70.

Pugh, G. (1989) Parents and professionals in pre-school services: Is partnership possible? In Wolfendale, S. (Ed.) *Parental Involvement: Developing Networks between School, Home and Community*. London: Cassell.

Quirk, R. (1972) *Speech Therapy Services*. London: HMSO.

Ramig, P., Bennett, E. (1995) Working with 7 to 12 year old children who stutter: Ideas for intervention in the public schools. *Language, Speech and Hearing Services in Schools*, **26**: 138–50.

RCSLT (1996) *Communicating Quality: Professional Standards for Speech and Language Therapists*. London: Royal College of Speech and Language Therapists.

RCSLT (1997) *The Role of the Speech and Language Therapist in the Multi-professional Assessment of Children with Special Education Needs*. London: Royal College of Speech and Language Therapists.

RCSLT (1998) *Response to 'Excellence for All' – DfEE Green Paper*. London: Royal College of Speech and Language Therapists.

Regina versus Lancashire County Council ex parte CM a minor (1989) *Family Law*: 395–6.

Reid, J., Millar, S., Tait, L., Donaldson, M.L., Dean, E.C., Thomson, G.O.B., Grieve, R. (1996) *The Role of the Speech and Language Therapist in the Education of Pupils with Special Educational Needs*. Edinburgh: Centre for Research in Child Development.

Rice, M., Wexler, K. (1996) Towards tense as a clinical marker of specific language impairment in English-speaking children. *Journal of Speech and Hearing Research*, **39**: 1239–57.

Robertson, A. (1983) Quest Screening, Diagnostic and Remediation Kit. Leeds: Arnold-Wheaton.

Robertson, S., Kersner, M., Davis, S. (1995) *A History of the College 1945–1995*. London: Royal College of Speech and Language Therapists.

Rosenberg, S., Curtiss, J. (1954) The effect of stuttering on the behaviour of the listener. *Journal of Abnormal Social Psychology*, 49: 355–61.

Roux, J. (1996) Working collaboratively with teachers: Supporting the newly qualified speech and language therapist in a mainstream school. *Child Language Teaching and Therapy*, 12: 48–59.

Ruscello, D., Lass, N., Schmitt, J., Pannbacker, M. (1994) Special educators' perceptions of stutterers. *Journal of Fluency Disorders*, 19: 125–32.

Ryan, B. (1984) Treatment of stuttering in school children. In Perkins, W.H. (Ed.) *Stuttering Disorders*, pp. 95–105. New York: Thieme-Stratton.

St Louis, K., Lass, N. (1981) A survey of communication disorders students' attitudes towards stuttering. *Journal of Fluency Disorders*, 6: 49–79.

Sallis, J. (1988) *Schools, Parents and Governors: A New Approach to Accountability*. London: Routledge.

Sayer, J. (1989) Facing issues in parents' responsibility for education. In Wolfendale, S. (Ed.) *Parental Involvement: Developing Networks Between School, Home and Community*. London: Cassell.

Schulz, H. (1977) Vergleichende Untersuchung von Sprachbehinderten und Nichtsprachbehinderten Schulern des 3. Schuljahres mit dem Rechentest DRE3 von Samstag, Sander und Schmidt. *Sprachheilarbeit*, 22: 86–95.

Seed, P. (1990) *Introducing Social Network Analysis in Social Work*. London: Jessica Kingsley.

Shaw, L., Luscombe M., Ostime, J. (1996) Collaborative Working in the Development of a School-based Speech and Language Therapy Service. Proceedings of the Golden Jubilee Conference, York: 1995, pp. 330–42. London: Royal College of Speech and Language Therapists.

Sheehan, J. (1975) Conflict theory and avoidance reduction therapy. In Eisenson, J. (Ed.) *Stuttering: A Second Symposium*. New York: Harper & Row.

SiLAS (1993) *Speech and Language Audit Software*. Glasgow: Mosaic.

Silverman, F., Marik, J. (1993) Teachers' perceptions of stuttering: A replication. *Language, Speech and Hearing Services in Schools*, 24: 108–9.

Sisson, E., Irving, A., Walton, A. (1994) Prioritising special needs. *Bulletin, Royal College of Speech and Language Therapists*, **December**: 5–6.

SOED (1991/93) *Curriculum and Assessment in Scotland – National Guidelines*. Edinburgh: Scottish Office Education Department.

SOED (1993) *Support for Learning – Staff Development Materials*. Dundee: Scottish Consultative Council on the Curriculum

SOEID (1994) *Effective Provision for Special Educational Needs*. Edinburgh: Scottish Office Education and Industry Department.

Stackhouse, J., Wells, B. (1997) *Children's Speech and Literacy Difficulties*. London: Whurr.

Stewart, T., Turnbull, J. (1995) *Working with Dysfluent Children*. Bicester: Winslow.

Stones, R. (1993) *Don't Pick on Me: How to Handle Bullying*. London: Piccadilly Press.

Taylor, A. (1997) Timetabling Therapist–Teacher Liaison Time within the Constraints of a Mainstream Primary School. Submitted in part-fulfilment of postgraduate award, Department of Speech and Language Therapy, University of Strathclyde.

Thomas, G. (1997) Inclusive schools for an inclusive society. *British Journal of Special Education*, 24: 103–7.

Tobin, M.J. (1998) Is blindness a handicap? *British Journal of Special Education*, 25: 107–13.

Topping, K. (1986) Which Parental Involvement in Reading Scheme? A Guide to Practitioners. *Paired Reading Bulletin*, 2 61–6.

Torgesen, J.K., Wagner, R.K., Rashotte, C.A. (1994) Longitudinal studies of phonological processing and reading. *Journal of Learning Disabilities*, **27**: 276–86.

Trevarthen, C., Aitken, K.J., Papoudi, D., Robarts, J.Z. (1996) *Children with Autism*. London: Jessica Kingsley.

Turnbull, A.P., Turnbull, H.R. (1986) *Families, Professionals and Exceptionality*. Columbus, OH: Merrill.

Van Riper, C. (1973) *The Treatment of Stuttering* Englewood Cliffs, NJ: Prentice Hall.

Visser, J. (1993) *Differentiation: Making It Work. Ideas for Staff Development*. Tamworth: National Association for Special Educational Needs.

Walker, M. (1976) *The Makaton Vocabulary*. Camberley: The Makaton Vocabulary Development Project.

Wedell, K. (1993) *Special Needs Education: The Next 25 Years*. London: National Commission on Education.

White, P., Collins, S. (1984) Stereotype formation by inference: A possible explanation for the 'stutterer' stereotype. *Journal of Speech and Hearing Research*, **27**: 567–70.

Williams, D., Melrose, B., Woods, C. (1969) The relationship between stuttering and academic achievement in children. *Journal of Communication Disorders*, **2**: 87–98.

Wing, L., Gould, J. (1979) Severe impairments of social interaction and associated abnormalities in children: Epidemiology and classification. *Journal of Autism and Developmental Disorders*, **9**: 11–29.

Wolfendale, S. (1983) *Parental Participation in Children's Development and Education*. London: Gordon and Brook.

Wolfendale, S. (1992) *Empowering Parents and Teachers: Working for Children*. London: Cassell.

Wolfensberger, W. (1972) *Normalisation*. Downsview, Ontario: National Institute on Mental Retardation.

Wolfensberger, W. (1995) Social rôle valorisation is too conservative. No, it is too radical. *Disability and Society*, **10**: 365–7.

Woods, C. (1978) Does the stigma shape the stutterer? *Journal of Communication Disorders*, **11**: 483–7.

Woods, C., Williams, D. (1976) Traits attributed to stuttering and normally fluent males. *Journal of Speech and Hearing Research*, **19**: 267–78.

Working Party of Scottish Principal Educational Psychologists (1988) Children with Communication Disorders. Unpublished mimeograph. Edinburgh: Moray House College of Education.

Wright, J., Graham, J. (1997) Where and when do speech and language therapists work with teachers? *British Journal of Special Education*, **24**: 171–4.

Yeakle, M., Cooper, E. (1986) Teacher perceptions of stuttering. *Journal of Fluency Disorders*, **11**: 345–59.

Index